D1413619

Atherosclerosis

A SCOPE® PUBLICATION

Antonio M. Gotto, Jr., MD, DPhil,
Consulting Author

Abel Lazzarini Robertson, Jr., MD, PhD

Stephen E. Epstein, MD

Michael E. DeBakey, MD,
and
Charles H. McCollum, III, MD

Herbert L. Gross
Editor

Larry L. Fites
Senior Art Director

Library of Congress Card Number 76-14368

Copyright ©1977. The Upjohn Company, Kalamazoo, Michigan 49001.

Reprinted 1979, 1980, 1983, 1985, 1988.

Printed in the United States of America

All rights reserved. No part of this book may be reproduced or transmitted in any form or by any means without written permission from the publisher.

8801-04R3

Contents

Introduction

Atherosclerosis is the most common disease that afflicts Western society. It is the underlying cause of most cardiovascular diseases, including myocardial infarctions and cerebrovascular insufficiency. The number of deaths related to cardiovascular disease in the United States is very nearly one million per year; more than one half of these are caused by coronary artery disease that is directly attributed to atherosclerosis.

This monograph is intended to provide the practicing physician (or physician-to-be) with a current view of research and treatment in the field of atherosclerosis. Each of the authors is both an investigator and a practitioner – each is involved not only in research but also with clinical problems on a daily basis. This dual role gives the authors a highly personal perspective which is reflected in the sections of the monograph. This monograph is, therefore, far more personal than a standard textbook and some of the concepts and interpretations are controversial. However, an effort was made to distinguish between information about which there is a general consensus and that which is still speculative.

The first section of the monograph considers the diagnosis and management of risk factors. In effect, it deals with the question so frequently asked by patients – "What can I do to prevent atherosclerosis?" – but emphasizes that we do not yet have a definitive, scientific experiment which establishes that reduction of risk factors can reduce cardiovascular mortality.

The second section reviews the pathogenesis of atherosclerosis. Because coronary artery disease is one of the most commonly encountered clinical manifestations of atherosclerosis, special emphasis is given to this condition. Other sections discuss the diagnosis of coronary artery disease and the medical treatment of stable angina pectoris. Finally, comprehensive consideration is given to surgical treatment, including a description of the various patterns and clinical presentations of atherosclerosis.

SECTION I

Diagnosis and Management of Risk Factors for Atherosclerosis

Antonio M. Gotto, Jr., MD, DPhil

The Bob and Vivian Smith Chairman
Department of Medicine
and
J.S. Abercrombie Professor
Departments of Medicine and Biochemistry
and
Scientific Director
National Heart and Blood Vessel Research
and Demonstration Center
Baylor College of Medicine
and
The Methodist Hospital
Houston, Texas

10

Risk Factor Hypothesis

The majority of people who die or are disabled because of atherosclerosis exhibit one or more identifiable characteristics called *risk factors*. Presumably, risk factors are present more frequently in people who develop atherosclerosis than in the general population. Estimates of the occurrence of major risk factors in individuals with atherosclerosis vary from 50% to 80%. The risk factor hypothesis is as follows: *if a person has a risk factor, he or she is more likely to develop clinical manifestations of atherosclerosis and is likely to do so earlier than is a person with no risk factors.*

If the hypothesis is valid, one would expect the atherosclerotic complications to be reduced if risk factors were corrected. This concept, however, has not been scientifically established. Several national studies are in progress to determine whether or not the correction of risk factors protects an individual from disability or premature death.

Primary Risk Factors

Risk factors for atherosclerosis are best defined in terms of coronary artery (Table I) and cerebrovascular diseases. The manifestations of coronary artery disease and angina pectoris are discussed in more detail in Sections II and III. Three primary risk factors that have been identified for premature coronary artery disease are hypercholesterolemia, hypertension, and smoking.

HYPERCHOLESTEROLEMIA

Hypercholesterolemia is a form of hyperlipidemia. By definition, hyperlipidemia is an elevation of plasma cholesterol levels or triglyceride concentrations, or both. Cholesterol is in the class of substances known as lipids. The cholesterol nucleus is a complex ring structure, and substances containing it are known as *steroids* or, if they contain a free alcohol, as *sterols* (Figure 1A). The average concentration of cholesterol in American adults ranges from 205 to 225 mg/100 ml. This value represents the concentration of total cholesterol, both esterified and unesterified or free. Approximately two thirds of the total cholesterol in plasma or serum is in the ester form (Figure 1A). Cholesterol and other plasma lipids are carried in the blood by emulsified, water-soluble forms called *plasma lipoproteins*. These are macromolecules containing cholesterol, cholesteryl ester, triglycerides, and phospholipids (Figure 1A). The lipoproteins contain protein components known as apoproteins or apolipoproteins. All lipid components are water insoluble; only when they are complexed with protein do they become water soluble. The cholesteryl esters and triglycerides are the least water soluble of the lipid components; the phospholipids are the most soluble; cholesterol is intermediate. The apoprotein and phospholipid constituents may function as detergents, or solubilizers, for the other components (Figure 1B).

Table I.
Treatable risk factors for coronary artery disease.

Primary:	Elevated serum cholesterol
	Elevated blood pressure
	Cigarette smoking
Secondary:	Elevated serum or plasma triglycerides
	Diabetes mellitus
	Obesity
	Lack of physical activity
	Stress: Type A personality

Figure 1A. Chemical structures of cholesterol, cholesteryl ester, phospholipid, and triglyceride.

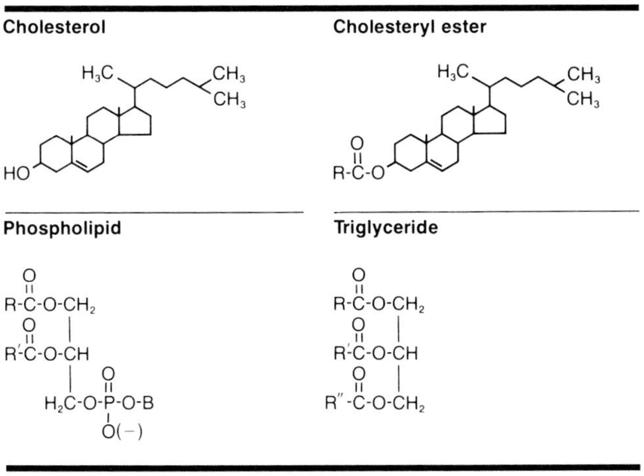

Cholesterol

Cholesteryl ester

Phospholipid

Triglyceride

R, R,́ R″ = Fatty acid   B = Base

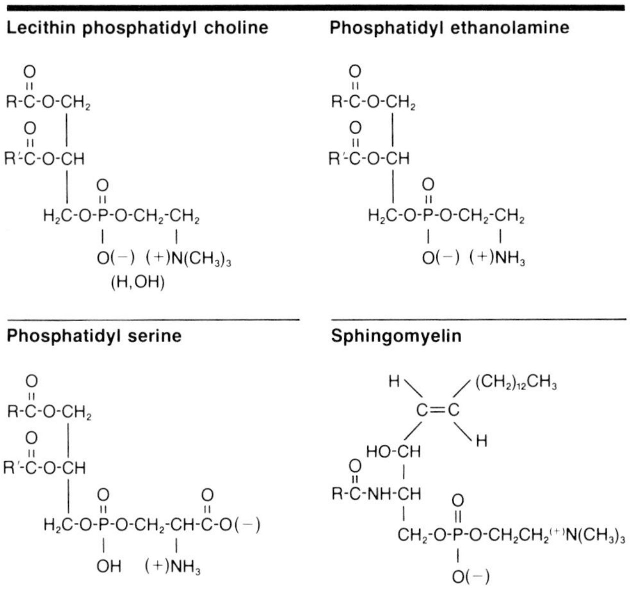

Lecithin phosphatidyl choline

Phosphatidyl ethanolamine

Phosphatidyl serine

Sphingomyelin

Figure 1B. Chemical structures of polar lipid molecules.

HYPERLIPOPROTEINEMIA

Gofman and his colleagues at the Donner Laboratory in Berkeley, California, were among the first to call attention to an association between high levels of plasma lipoproteins and an increased incidence of clinical atherosclerosis. Hyperlipidemia, when classified on the basis of individual lipoprotein families, is called *hyperlipoproteinemia*. These investigators developed an *atherosclerosis index*, which is based on the profile of plasma lipoproteins. Most of their work focused on the use of the analytical ultracentrifuge.

Ultracentrifugal characteristics and electrophoretic migration are the primary means for separating and classifying the different families or classes of plasma lipoproteins. Each lipoprotein family forms discrete particles of characteristic, though not fixed, lipid and protein composition; these particles appear spherically shaped when viewed with the electron microscope (Figure 2A). Five families may be identified: (1) chylomicron, (2) very-low-density lipoprotein (VLDL), (3) intermediate-density lipoprotein (IDL), (4) low-density

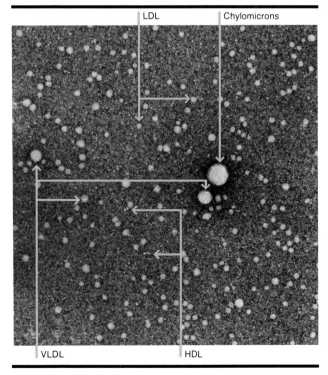

Figure 2A. Electron microscopic view of the families of lipoproteins.

12

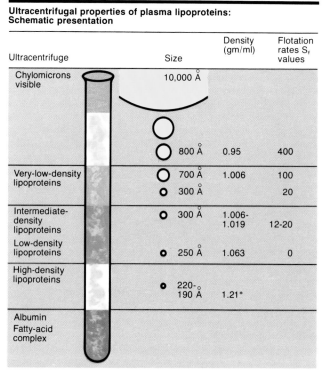

Figure 2B. Schematic representation of ultracentrifugal properties of plasma lipoproteins.

Ultracentrifugal properties of plasma lipoproteins: Schematic presentation

Ultracentrifuge	Size	Density (gm/ml)	Flotation rates S_f values
Chylomicrons visible	10,000 Å		
	800 Å	0.95	400
Very-low-density lipoproteins	700 Å	1.006	100
	300 Å		20
Intermediate-density lipoproteins	300 Å	1.006-1.019	12-20
Low-density lipoproteins	250 Å	1.063	0
High-density lipoproteins	220-190 Å	1.21*	
Albumin Fatty-acid complex			

*The 1.21 infranatant may also contain varied amounts of apoA-I, lysolecithin, and small quantities of other apoproteins and lipids.

lipoprotein (LDL), and (5) high-density lipoprotein (HDL) (Table II).

Lipoproteins differ in size, density (Figure 2B), ultracentrifugal properties, and electrophoretic characteristics. The smaller the lipoprotein particle, the greater its protein content and density. Thus, chylomicrons have the fastest ultracentrifugal flotation rates, whereas HDL have the slowest. On paper and agarose-gel electrophoresis, chylomicrons do not leave the origin, while the VLDL migrate just beyond β-globulins; the latter are referred to as the pre-β-lipoproteins (Figure 3). Since LDL migrate with the β-globulins, they are referred to as the β-lipoproteins. The IDL have intermediate mobility between the LDL and VLDL. HDL are called the α-lipoprotein, owing to their co-migration with the α-globulin family. Because of their lipid content, lipoproteins have lower densities than do other plasma proteins. Therefore, they float at densities at which other plasma proteins sink or sediment, eg, less than 1.210 gm/ml. When the rate of flotation is measured under certain standard conditions, the value is referred to as the S_f.

Each family of lipoproteins performs different functions in the body. For example, chylomicrons transport most of the dietary constituents, while VLDL carry most of the triglycerides. Approximately 60% of plasma cholesterol is carried by LDL. HDL appear to serve as a reservoir for small apoproteins involved in triglyceride transport; they also are the major plasma source of an apoprotein activator required to esterify cholesterol. For some reason, HDL levels tend to be higher in women than in men. It may be that HDL act as a vehicle for transporting cholesterol from tissues back to the liver, possibly protecting women against the development of atherosclerosis. There is no direct evidence for this theory. However, epidemiological evidence suggests that high levels of HDL may protect one from coronary artery disease.

Diagnosis of Hyperlipidemia and Hyperlipoproteinemia
Using paper electrophoresis of plasma lipoproteins and plasma lipid estimations as a basis, Fredrickson, Levy, and Lees at the National Heart Institute proposed a system for classifying the hyperlipoproteinemias or hyperlipidemias. The classification system is based primarily on which family of plasma lipoproteins is elevated (Table III). Thus, in type I, chylomicrons and, concomitantly, triglycerides are markedly increased. In normal subjects, under ordinary circumstances, detectable chylomicrons should not be present after

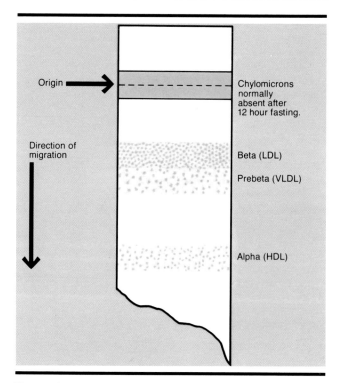

Figure 3. Paper electrophoresis patterns for normal fasting lipoproteins.

Table II.
Properties of the five lipoprotein families.

Lipoprotein family	Electrophoresis (paper or agarose gel)	Ultracentrifugation
Chylomicrons	Nonmigrating	Density* less than 0.95
VLDL	Pre-β mobility	Density 0.95-1.006 S_f 20-400
IDL	Pre-β to β mobility	Density 1.006-1.019 S_f 12-20
LDL	β mobility	Density 1.019-1.063 S_f 0-12
HDL HDL$_2$ HDL$_3$	α mobility	Density 1.063-1.210

*Density value is measured in gm/ml.

the individual has fasted for 12 hours. In type IIa, concentrations of LDL and cholesterol are high. In type IIb, LDL, cholesterol, VLDL, and triglycerides are all increased. Type III is associated with the occurrence of an abnormal lipoprotein which has β-electrophoretic mobility but which floats in VLDL because of its high content of triglyceride. Type IV is characterized by an increase in VLDL concentrations. In type V, chylomicrons are present and the VLDL level is increased.

Table III.
Classification system for the hyperlipoproteinemias.

Phenotype	Definition	Dietary management	Drugs
Type I	Hyperchylomicronemia* + absolute deficiency of LPL or PHLA	1. Restriction of fat to about 35 gm/day 2. Supplementation with medium-chain triglycerides	None effective at present
Type IIa	↑ LDL or β-lipoproteins	1. Low-cholesterol diet (less than 300 mg/day) 2. Decreased intake of saturated fats 3. Increased intake of polyunsaturated fats	1. Cholestyramine, 16-24 gm/day 2. Nicotinic acid, 3 gm/day 3. D-thyroxine, 2-6 mg/day†
Type IIb	↑ LDL or β-lipoproteins and ↑ VLDL or pre-β-lipoproteins	1. Reduction to ideal body weight 2. Low-cholesterol diet (less than 300 mg/day) 3. Decreased intake of saturated fats 4. Increased intake of polyunsaturated fats	1. Cholestyramine, 16-24 gm/day 2. Nicotinic acid, 3 gm/day
Type III	Floating β-lipoprotein	1. Reduction to ideal body weight 2. Low-cholesterol diet (less than 300 mg/day) 3. Decreased intake of saturated fat	1. Clofibrate, 2 gm/day
Type IV	↑ VLDL or pre-β-lipoproteins	1. Reduction to ideal body weight 2. Carbohydrate restricted to 40% of calories 3. Substitute polyunsaturated fats for saturated fats 4. Restrict alcohol to two servings daily 5. Cholesterol intake 300-400 mg/day	1. Clofibrate, 2 gm/day 2. Nicotinic acid, 3 gm/day
Type V	Hyperchylomicronemia and ↑ VLDL or pre-β-lipoproteins, LPL, or PHLA present	1. Reduction to ideal body weight 2. Reduction of fat to 30% of daily calories 3. Alcohol not recommended 4. Increased intake of protein 5. Cholesterol intake 300-400 mg/day	1. Nicotinic acid, 3 gm/day 2. Norethindrone acetate, 2.5-5.0 mg/day‡ 3. Oxandrolone, 2.5 mg t.i.d.‡

* These definitions must be established by cholesterol, triglyceride, and lipoprotein determinations on plasma or serum obtained after a 12-hour fast. The subject should have a stable weight, be on a regular diet, not be acutely ill; and not be taking lipid-lowering drugs when tested.

† Should be used with caution in view of reports by Coronary Drug Project, JAMA 220:996-1008, 1972. Contraindicated in patients with coronary artery disease or cardiac arrhythmia.
‡ Investigational drug for treating hyperlipidemia or HLP.

The first step in detecting hyperlipidemia is to measure the concentration of serum or plasma lipids, specifically cholesterol and triglyceride. A blood sample should be obtained from the patient after he has fasted for 12 hours. At the time of the sampling, the patient's condition is important; for example, if he or she is recovering from an acute myocardial infarction, the cholesterol and LDL levels are likely to be depressed and levels of VLDL and triglyceride increased. This is probably a consequence of stress and does not reflect the true baseline condition. Ideally, when the plasma lipid and lipoprotein levels are analyzed, the patient should be in good health, on a regular diet, and not taking medication that would affect the tests. A number of other variables may affect plasma cholesterol values; seasonal fluctuations are a good example. Also, cholesterol may be decreased by as much as 10% by having the patient recline for a period of time before the test. This is due to an increase in plasma volume. Additional uncertainties are caused by differences in methodology in lipid measurement from one laboratory to another. For example, when cholesterol is measured directly from whole blood by an SMA-12 procedure, the value is 10% to 15% higher than that measured in a sample using the standard Abell-Kendall method.

There is no precise definition of hypercholesterolemia or hypertriglyceridemia. Table IV provides a list of the values currently used at The Methodist Hospital Lipid Clinic. In this clinic, if an adult patient has a cholesterol level over 265 mg/100 ml, we believe further medical evaluation is indicated. In a younger person, a value as low as 220 mg/100 ml might require further evaluation. These values should not be considered exact guidelines, but rather arbitrary cutoffs for defining overt hyperlipidemia in the United States. Evidence from several studies shows that the serum or plasma cholesterol is a continuous risk factor for coronary heart disease. It has not been possible to define a single cutoff point to separate those people at risk from those who are not. Dr. Irving Wright, speaking on behalf of the Inter-Society Commission for Heart Disease Resources, has pointed out that most cholesterol values are given to the physician and patient in the context of a *statistically normal* or acceptable level. This group believes that 240 mg/100 ml should be considered as the uppermost acceptable value for adults. The so-called normal value is higher than the optimal or desirable value, which should probably range from 150 to 180 mg/100 ml.

During the patient's medical workup, a secondary cause for the hyperlipidemia may be uncovered (Table V). Personal and medical family history, a physical examination, and laboratory tests to exclude secondary causes are then in order. If secondary causes can be eliminated, the type of underlying primary hyperlipidemia should be identified. As previously mentioned, the first step is measurement of a fasting patient's plasma cholesterol and triglyceride concentrations. Another useful step is the observation of plasma or serum after cold storage for 8 to 12 hours (Figure 4). Normal plasma contains detectable quantities of VLDL, LDL, and HDL, but does not contain chylomicrons. Also it will appear clear to the naked eye. After cold storage, chylomicrons, if present, emerge as a creamy layer at the top of the tube. This may indicate either that the patient is not fasting or that hyperlipidemia is present in the form of type I, V, or even type III. Elevations of LDL and cholesterol, per se, do not cause the plasma to appear turbid. However, plasma triglyceride concentrations greater than about 400 mg/100 ml usually cause turbidity.

It is important to determine which pattern or phenotype of hyperlipidemia is present in the patient, because of the different syndromes associated with each pattern. A given pattern tends to be inherited within a family, resulting in *familial hyperlipidemia*. However, the particular variety of genetic hyperlipidemia that is present cannot be diagnosed from the lipoprotein pattern, or phenotype, which is actually a laboratory designation. More than one phenotype may be present in a particular family. The lipoprotein pattern makes it possible to arrive at a more rational basis for treatment. The lipoprotein pattern is called the *phenotype*, as distinct from the *genotype*. The latter cannot be determined from the phenotype. Classical patterns of familial hyperlipidemia probably are not the most common forms of hyperlipidemia that predispose a person to atherosclerosis. However, when hyperlipidemia is present, it is important to identify other family members who also may be affected.

If a phenotype is not apparent from measurements of cholesterol and triglyceride levels, from plasma examination, or from the medical history and physical examination, then the concentrations of plasma lipoproteins must be measured. Electrophoresis is the most frequently used method (Figure 4) for measurement. There are several types of electrophoresis, but almost all of those used in clinical laboratories are qualitative or only semiquantitative. If both the cholesterol and triglyceride values are elevated, or if the cholesterol value is in the borderline range (from 250 to 280 mg/100 ml), then it is

Figure 4. Laboratory findings in a patient with hyperlipoproteinemia.

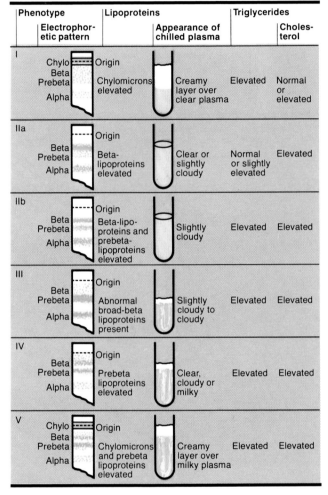

Phenotype		Lipoproteins		Triglycerides	
	Electrophoretic pattern		Appearance of chilled plasma		Cholesterol
I	Chylo / Beta / Prebeta / Alpha	Origin / Chylomicrons elevated	Creamy layer over clear plasma	Elevated	Normal or elevated
IIa	Beta / Prebeta / Alpha	Origin / Beta-lipoproteins elevated	Clear or slightly cloudy	Normal or slightly elevated	Elevated
IIb	Beta / Prebeta / Alpha	Origin / Beta-lipoproteins and prebeta-lipoproteins elevated	Slightly cloudy	Elevated	Elevated
III	Beta / Prebeta / Alpha	Origin / Abnormal broad-beta lipoproteins present	Slightly cloudy to cloudy	Elevated	Elevated
IV	Beta / Prebeta / Alpha	Origin / Prebeta lipoproteins elevated	Clear, cloudy or milky	Elevated	Elevated
V	Chylo / Beta / Prebeta / Alpha	Origin / Chylomicrons and prebeta lipoproteins elevated	Creamy layer over milky plasma	Elevated	Elevated

Table IV.
Cutoff values for defining overt hyperlipidemia.*

Age	Cholesterol	Triglycerides
1-9	200	120
10-19	205	140
20-29	210	140
30-39	240	150
40-49	265	160
>50	265	190

* These values should not be considered as optimal or desirable levels. We do not know what a "normal" or "safe" cholesterol or triglyceride concentration is at the present time. The best available evidence is that the cholesterol concentration has a continuous relationship with the risk of coronary artery disease or myocardial infarction.

Table V.
Secondary causes of hyperlipoproteinemia.

Hypothyroidism	Obstructive liver disease
Diabetes mellitus	Pancreatitis
Nephrotic syndrome	Dysglobulinemia
Renal failure (uremia)	Glycogen storage disease
Alcoholism	Porphyria

Table VI.
Simplified method for estimating LDL-cholesterol.**

Plasma cholesterol =	LDL-cholesterol + VLDL-cholesterol + HDL-cholesterol
Require:	Chylomicrons absent
	Floating β-lipoprotein absent
	Triglycerides less than 400 mg/100 ml
Measure:	Plasma cholesterol directly
	Plasma triglyceride
	Cholesterol not precipitated by heparin and manganese
Assume:	Cholesterol not precipitated by heparin and manganese = HDL-cholesterol
	VLDL-cholesterol = plasma triglyceride/5
	LDL-cholesterol = plasma cholesterol − plasma triglyceride/5 − HDL-cholesterol

**Adapted from Friedwald, Levy, and Fredrickson.

necessary to measure LDL or LDL-cholesterol concentration in order to diagnose or exclude type II hyperlipidemia. Some patients, particularly women, have normal LDL concentrations despite cholesterol levels as high as 300 mg/100 ml. The high cholesterol concentration in these women is due to an increased concentration of HDL, a condition not considered pathological.

Friedwald, Levy, and Fredrickson have suggested a method for estimating LDL-cholesterol without using the ultracentrifuge (Table VI). This method cannot be applied if (1) type III hyperlipidemia is present, (2) chylomicronemia is present after fasting, or (3) the triglyceride concentration is over 400 mg/100 ml. Special tests are needed to diagnose type III hyperlipidemia. One such test, performed in the preparative ultracentrifuge in conjunction with electrophoresis, determines whether a lipoprotein with β-electrophoretic mobility floats at the normal plasma density of 1.006 gm/ml. A second test is based on the ratio of VLDL-cholesterol to VLDL or plasma triglyceride.

Primary hyperlipidemia may be sporadic or familial. In a University of Washington study of the occurrence of hyperlipidemia in the relatives of myocardial infarction survivors, it was estimated that about one third had some form of familial hyperlipidemia. In this study, three important monogenic or dominant inherited disorders were described: (1) familial hypertriglyceridemia, (2) familial hypercholesterolemia, and (3) familial combined hyperlipidemia. Geneticists in Seattle presented evidence that each of these disorders was inherited as a monogenic dominant trait. However, other geneticists have disputed certain of these interpretations, and a consensus of opinion is not yet available.

A brief definition of the lipoprotein phenotypes (Table III) and their clinical features is given to help the physician diagnose these disorders and prescribe appropriate modes of therapy. The information presented previously concerning the individual lipoprotein classes is important because these findings are most commonly used to define hyperlipoproteinemia. Ordinarily, chylomicrons should not be present in detectable quantities after an overnight fast by the patient. In type I there is significant chylomicronemia. However, the presence of chylomicrons after fasting is not absolutely specific for type I because this condition, by definition, is present in type V and may also be a feature of untreated type III.

Characteristic of type I is a total deficiency of a chylomicron-lowering agent found in the adipose tissue, identified as lipoprotein lipase. Since lipoprotein lipase is released into plasma following the intravenous administration of heparin, it is called *postheparin lipolytic activity* (PHLA). The activity is due to a triglyceride lipase, which catalyzes the hydrolysis of triglycerides in lipoproteins or in artificial emulsions. In normal subjects, PHLA or triglyceride lipase is present in adipose tissue and differs from a hepatic lipase in two respects: (1) in apoprotein requirements for activation, and (2) in inhibition by protamine sulfate and high salt concentration. Both adipose tissue and hepatic activities are released by intravenous injection of heparin. Little, if any, detectable PHLA is found in the patient's circulation after normal fasting conditions. Following heparin administration, small quantities of the hepatic activity may appear in the plasma of some patients with type I, but the adipose-tissue activity is absent.

Measurement of postheparin lipolytic activity is complicated and unsatisfactory. A relatively simple all-or-none test may be performed by determining if there is an increase in the electrophoretic mobility of the plasma lipoproteins after heparin injection. Such an increase excludes the diagnosis of type I. The increased mobility is due to the release of large quantities of unesterified fatty acid after triglyceride hydrolysis. Secondary causes of type I include diabetic acidosis, myxedema, and dysglobulinemia associated with a heparin-binding globulin. In the latter situation, an injection of a larger-than-usual amount of heparin may overcome the inhibition.

As chylomicrons and VLDL circulate through peripheral tissues, their triglyceride components are partially hydrolized and depleted (Figure 5A). The resulting cholesteryl-ester-enriched particle is referred to as a remnant. In man, the chylomicron remnants are rapidly removed by the liver, whereas VLDL remnants are believed to be converted largely to LDL (Figure 5B). There is some evidence in experimental animals that remnants may be preferentially taken up by arterial smooth-muscle cells, which would give these partially degraded lipoproteins a potential role in the etiology of arteriosclerosis.

Familial type I is extremely rare and almost always appears in childhood. *Eruptive xanthomas* appear as red maculopapules, usually on the face, buttocks, and mucous membranes. These are due to a severely elevated concentration of plasma triglycerides. Hepatosplenomegaly is present because of lipid deposition in the reticuloendothelial system. The plasma is creamy white from the hypertriglyceridemia (triglyceride elevation in the thousands). This may cause *lipemia retinalis*, a condition characterized by a whitish appearance of the retinal arterioles. Interestingly, despite the marked elevation of serum lipids, early arteriosclerosis is not known to be associated with this phenotype.

Type II hyperlipidemia is defined by an increase in the concentration of LDL or LDL-cholesterol. If there is accompanying endogenous hypertriglyceridemia, that is, if VLDL concentrations are elevated, then the pattern is type IIb; otherwise it is type IIa. Hypothyroidism and nephrosis are secondary conditions that may produce the type II pattern.

Figure 5A. Phases of chylomicron metabolism: (1) intestinal synthesis, (2) hydrolysis of triglyceride in peripheral tissues to form remnants, (3) hepatic removal of remnants.

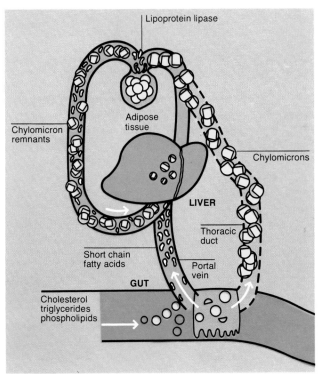

◎ Chylomicron 700-1000 Å
◉ Chylomicron remnants
◊ FFA

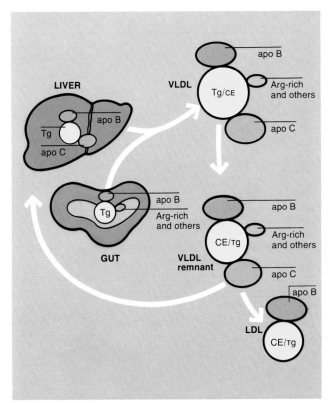

FIGURE 5B. Synthesis of VLDL and conversion of VLDL remnants to LDL. In some species (such as the rat), the major metabolism of the VLDL remnant is via the liver; in man, the major pathway seems to be to LDL.

The best-known inherited hyperlipidemia in which type II occurs is familial hypercholesterolemia. The phenotype is usually IIa, although IIb is not uncommon. Familial hypercholesterolemia is perhaps the most extensively studied of the genetically determined hyperlipidemias. The features most typical of this classical disorder are (1) an association with a high incidence of premature arteriosclerosis and (2) a mean age of myocardial infarction onset in men from 41 to 44 years — women, in comparison, are protected approximately 10 to 15 years longer.

Classical familial hypercholesterolemia appears most frequently to be inherited as a monogenic dominant trait, occurring as often as one in 500 in the general population. Heterozygotes are common, but homozygotes are rare. Screening the first-degree relatives of the patient (heterozygote) is important, because one of his parents and statistically one half of his siblings and offspring are affected.

In the heterozygote, the findings of *xanthelasma* (Figure 6A, lipid plaques) on the eyelids, *tendinous xanthoma* (Figure 6B), or *corneal arcus* (Figure 6C), and clinical evidence of atherosclerosis usually do not appear until adulthood. By contrast, the child who inherits the trait from both parents (the homozygote) develops skin lesions, yellowish xanthomas not attached to tendons, and corneal arcus in the first few years of life. Such patients are often affected by severe atherosclerosis by the time they reach their teens. Homozygotes (Figure 6D) usually die in childhood of severe coronary artery disease, often of a cardiac arrhythmia. The most useful diagnostic criterion for familial hypercholesterolemia is an elevation of LDL or LDL-cholesterol early in life. In some instances, the chemical changes may be detected even in umbilical cord blood.

From the previous discussion, it is apparent, then, that until adulthood, the usual heterozygote patient with familial hypercholesterolemia has hypercholesterolemia and hyperbetalipoproteinemia (ie, an increase in LDL) as the only identifying features. Recently, Brown and Goldstein have observed that a specific cell receptor for LDL is absent (Figure 7) or defective in tissue-culture fibroblasts from homozygotes with familial hypercholesterolemia. In these studies, heterozygotes showed an intermediate defect in which about 40% of the normal receptors were reported to be present. Ordinarily, in tissue culture the intracellular synthesis of cholesterol is related inversely to the cholesterol concentration in the medium. When cholesterol is presented to the abnormal

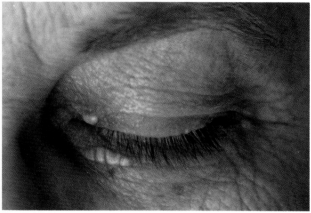

Figure 6A. Xanthelasma or lipid plaques on the eyelids of the heterozygote with familial hypercholesterolemia.

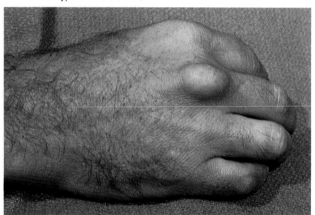

Figure 6B. Tendinous xanthoma in the heterozygote with familial hypercholesterolemia.

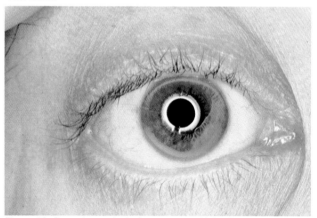

Figure 6C. Corneal arcus in the heterozygote with familial hypercholesterolemia.

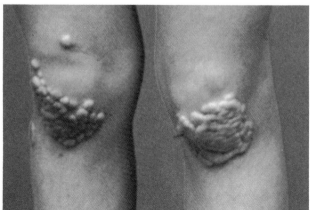

Figure 6D. Typical xanthoma in homozygote with familial hypercholesterolemia.

cell in the form of LDL, the extracellular cholesterol is less effective in shutting off cholesterol synthesis by the cell. Because the cell receptor for LDL is absent, the LDL-cholesterol is unable to gain entry into the cell. Consequently, for a given extracellular LDL concentration, the abnormal fibroblast makes too much cholesterol. This is due to an inability to suppress hydroxymethylglutaryl coenzyme A (HMG CoA) reductase, the rate-limiting enzyme in cholesterol biosynthesis (Figure 7). There is also a decrease in LDL degradation and intracellular cholesterol esterification.

The physiological significance of the specific receptor for LDL remains to be established. At present, however, there is no evidence that such a receptor exists in the liver. Evidence to date suggests that chylomicron remnants are the plasma lipoprotein intermediates most efficient in suppressing cholesterol synthesis by the liver. Animal studies have suggested that LDL catabolism occurs primarily in peripheral tissues. If this is correct, the specific LDL receptor identified in fibroblasts might play a significant role in LDL degradation (Figure 7). A defective receptor, or a deficiency in the number of receptors, could lead to a slower catabolism of LDL by peripheral tissues. The result would be the requirement of a higher circulating level of LDL to saturate the existing receptors. At a given LDL concentration, less lipoprotein would be bound to the cell and degraded by the mutant cell. Similarly, there would be less suppression of intracellular cholesterol synthesis. Several investigators have identified persons with clinical features characteristic of homozygous familial hypercholesterolemia who have only a partial defect in the LDL receptor, similar to that of the heterozygotes. Also, in one patient with typical clinical features of a homozygote, the fibroblasts were able to bind LDL but could not internalize it.

Fogelman, Popjak, et al have introduced the alternative view that the major cellular defect in patients with familial hypercholesterolemia is the inability to retain intracellular cholesterol. Thus, an increased synthesis of cholesterol by the cell is viewed as a compensatory response to an increase in cellular cholesterol loss. Further work is required to relate more precisely the intracellular defect of LDL and cholesterol metabolism in familial hypercholesterolemia to the clinical manifestations of this disorder.

To summarize, the presumed sequence of events in LDL catabolism by peripheral tissues is as follows: LDL is bound to a specific cell receptor; the LDL is internalized by endocytosis from the vesicles to the lysosomes, where degradation

Figure 7. LDL and cholesterol metabolism in skin fibroblasts of homozygotes with familial hyper-cholesterolemia.

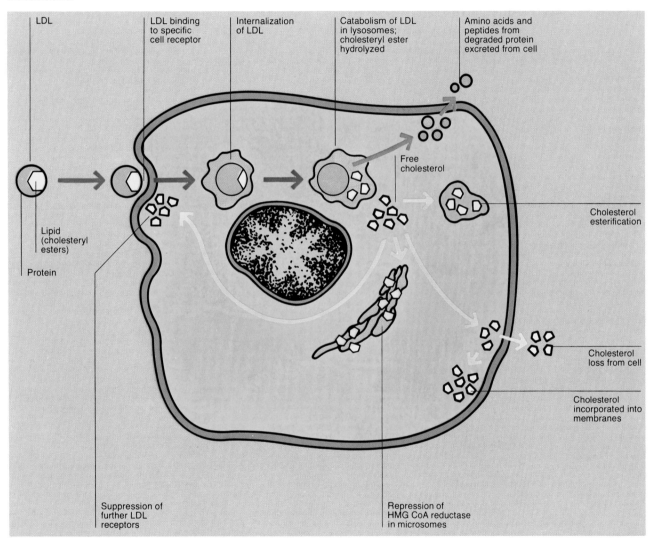

of LDL protein and cholesteryl ester occurs. The amino acids and peptides from the degraded protein are then excreted extracellularly, while the free cholesterol causes the intracellular repression of HMG CoA reductase formation, an increase in cholesterol esterification, and a suppression of further LDL receptors (Figure 7).

There are a limited number of ways in which the peripheral cell can dispose of excess intracellular cholesterol. Choles-terol may be esterified in peripheral tissues, but the cell probably has a limited capacity for storing cholesteryl esters. Alternatively, the cholesterol may be incorporated into the cell membrane. If this occurs, there probably is a concomitant increase in phospholipid synthesis because of the careful balance between the ratio of cholesterol and phospholipid in the cell membranes. Lastly, the cholesterol can be excreted from the cell, from where it would presumably be transported to the liver. The liver excretes cholesterol in the bile as a neutral steroid or converts it to a bile acid, which then can be excreted.

The total daily turnover of cholesterol by the average adult is approximately 1 gm. Cholesterol cannot be catabolized or broken down by peripheral tissues. If it is correct that peripheral tissues are the primary sites for LDL degradation, then the body must possess some mechanism for transporting cholesterol from these sites back to the liver.

Glomset suggested that HDL is one of the potential cholesterol carriers. HDL apoproteins combined with phospholipids have been shown to interact with cells and to promote cholesterol removal. It is not known if this occurs in the intact organism. The enzyme lecithin cholesterol acyltransferase (LCAT) catalyzes cholesterol esterification in the blood and requires one of the HDL apoproteins for activation. In the HDL-LCAT model of cholesterol transfer, the free sterol is removed from cells, transported in HDL, and esterified through the influence of LCAT. Whether other lipoprotein families serve as intermediaries between HDL and the liver is not known.

Arteries, including the aorta and the coronary vessels, are believed to have only very limited ability to synthesize cholesterol. Most of the cholesterol accumulating in the arteries must be derived from the blood, where it is carried by the plasma lipoproteins. However, it is conceivable that under certain aberrant conditions, faulty regulation of cholesterol synthesis by the smooth-muscle cells of the arterial wall could contribute to the pathogenesis of arteriosclerosis (see Section II). Brown and Goldstein have suggested such a possibility in familial hypercholesterolemia, but this hypothesis is speculative.

Familial combined hyperlipidemia also has been associated with coronary artery disease. The lipoprotein pattern is usually type IIb. However, in certain individuals, a type IV or even type IIa phenotype has been described. Tendinous xanthoma occurs less frequently than when familial hypercholesterolemia is present. Perhaps the most characteristic distinction between these disorders is that familial hypercholesterolemia occurs in childhood, whereas familial combined hyperlipidemia usually cannot be diagnosed until early adulthood.

Type III hyperlipidemia is often of familial etiology, although an association with hypothyroidism has been reported. Familial type III appears clinically distinct from familial hypercholesterolemia in a number of ways. It is less common

and the hyperlipidemia does not usually appear until adulthood. It is not known whether the floating or abnormal β-lipoprotein is actually present in childhood, but hyperlipidemia per se (hypercholesterolemia or hypertriglyceridemia) can be detected. Although coronary and peripheral atherosclerosis may be present, the cutaneous manifestations differ from those of familial hypercholesterolemia in that the lesions are usually tuberous and not attached to tendons (Figure 8A). Some patients with familial hypercholesterolemia, however, may also have tuberous lesions as a prominent feature (Figure 8B). A planar or palmar xanthoma (Figure 8C) is a lesion highly characteristic of type III hyperlipidemia. This lesion results from the deposition of lipid in the palmar creases of the hands.

Biochemically, type III hyperlipidemia is usually defined by the presence of an abnormal β-lipoprotein (*floating beta*), because of its typical properties in the standard ultracentrifuge, or *broad-beta* lipoprotein for its electrophoretic characteristics. Occurrence of the type III pattern within a kindred is called familial broad-beta disease. The abnormal lipoprotein contains an unusually rich complement of triglyceride, resulting in isolation at a density less than 1.006 gm/ml (VLDL range). When ultracentrifugation is performed in the usual angle-head rotor, the electrophoretic pattern is a rather wide, poorly defined beta band. The presence of a β-lipoprotein in the VLDL range causes increases in the ratio of VLDL-cholesterol to triglyceride in the VLDL. A ratio of VLDL-cholesterol to plasma triglycerides greater than 0.30 may be used as a criterion for defining the type III phenotype in patients with hypertriglyceridemia. By using rate zonal ultracentrifugation, the abnormal lipoprotein may be completely separated from VLDL. It has a density of 1.006 to 1.019 gm/ml, is referred to as LP-III, and is very similar to the *intermediate-density lipoprotein*. Ultracentrifugation with electrophoresis, cholesterol, and triglyceride measurements are necessary to establish this diagnosis. Some evidence indicates that the VLDL in type III contain increased amounts of a protein referred to as *arginine-rich protein*, because of its high arginine content. A similar increase in arginine-rich protein has been described in patients with hypothyroidism. Increased levels of an analogous protein have been observed in animals after cholesterol feeding. The significance of the arginine-rich protein in cholesterol transport is potentially great, but is not understood at present.

Type IV hyperlipidemia is defined by an increase in

Figure 8A. Tuberous unattached xanthomas in type III hyperlipidemia.

Figure 8C. Planar or palmar xanthoma, a deposition of lipid in the palmar creases of the hands, in type III hyperlipidemia.

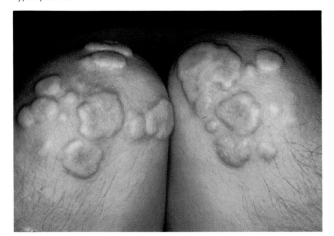

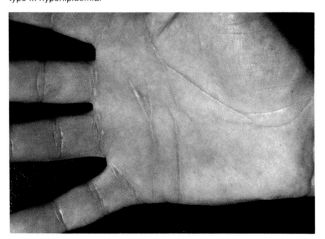

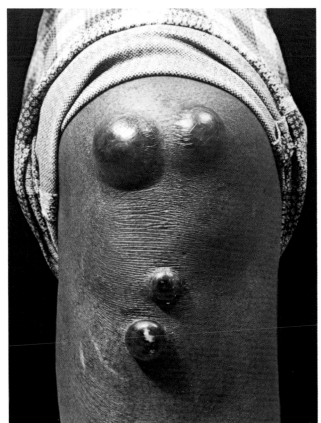

Figure 8B. Tuberous xanthomas in type III hyperlipidemia.

VLDL, the absence of chylomicrons and floating β-lipoprotein, and a normal concentration of LDL. Another name for this condition is *endogenous hypertriglyceridemia*. It is the most commonly encountered form of hyperlipidemia in the American population. Depending upon the cutoff point established for plasma triglycerides, 15% to 25% of the adult population may be affected. Obesity, a high intake of alcohol, and perhaps a high consumption of simple sugars, exacerbate endogenous hypertriglyceridemia. An association between coronary artery disease and type IV hyperlipidemia has been described. Since arteriosclerosis and endogenous hypertriglyceridemia occur so frequently in Americans, it is difficult to establish a cause-and-effect relationship. In one study, genetic analysis suggested that familial hypertriglyceridemia (type IV) was the most commonly inherited form of hyperlipidemia in the relatives of myocardial infarction survivors. In another study of patients with familial type IV at the National Heart, Lung and Blood Institute (NHLBI), secretion of insulin was normal in about a third of the group, high in a third, and low in a third. Apparently diabetes mellitus, uremia, and pancreatitis can mimic primary endogenous hypertriglyceridemia.

Type V hyperlipidemia is defined by the presence of chylomicronemia after fasting and by an increased concentration of VLDL. Usually, the level of PHLA or of adipose-tissue lipase is depressed. In contrast to familial type I (which appears in childhood), familial type V occurs only in adults. To further distinguish type V from type I, the clinician must determine whether detectable triglyceride lipase activity is present in adipose tissue. Clinical features of type V include the following: (1) recurrent bouts of abdominal pain, associated with a worsening of the hypertriglyceridemia, (2) acute and chronic pancreatitis, (3) an abnormal glucose tolerance test, (4) hyperuricemia, (5) hepatosplenomegaly, and (6) occasionally eruptive xanthomas on the skin resembling those occurring in type I (Figure 8D).

In summary, to evaluate the nature of a patient's hyperlipidemia (Table VII), the physician must first determine the phenotype. For this, he must have measurements of plasma cholesterol and triglyceride after the patient has fasted. The physician should also observe the plasma after storage, obtain a careful medical and family history from the patient, perform a physical examination, and measure the concentration of plasma lipoproteins by electrophoresis. After the phenotype is determined, secondary causes should be excluded before establishing the diagnosis of primary hyperlipidemia. Finally, prior to the consideration of treatment, in order to determine whether the condition is sporadic or familial, the patient's first-degree relatives must be screened.

Treatment should be considered in the context of present knowledge of the various phenotypes of hyperlipidemia and arteriosclerosis. The finding of familial type II or familial hypercholesterolemia is a very important predisposing factor for premature coronary artery disease. The same appears to be true of familial combined hyperlipidemia, which most often appears as a type IIb pattern. Based on current evidence, coronary artery disease and peripheral arteriosclerosis appear to accompany type III. However, the relatively small number of subjects studied to date precludes a more definitive correlation. The association of type IV with coronary and peripheral arteriosclerosis is uncertain, although there are numerous published reports describing such a correlation. We believe that an association may exist in some individuals, families, or in certain populations. Perhaps other risk factors (hypertension, cigarette smoking, diabetes, obesity, or an excessive consumption of alcohol) work in conjunction with the endogenous hypertriglyceridemia to promote arteriosclerosis. The relationship between type V and atherosclerosis is also uncertain. Available but inconclusive data suggest that there is a stronger association with peripheral atherosclerosis than with coronary disease.

We suspect that overt hyperlipidemia in the United States, as it is usually defined, affects a minority of patients with clinical evidence of atherosclerosis. At The Methodist Hospi-

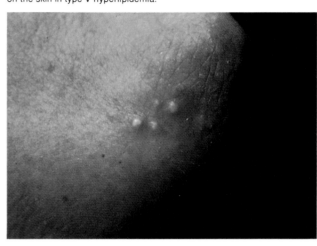

Figure 8D. Eruptive xanthomas occasionally found on the skin in type V hyperlipidemia.

Table VII.
Workup of a patient with hyperlipoproteinemia.

Detection	Elevated plasma cholesterol or triglyceride or both
Establish Phenotype	Medical and family history
	Physical examination
	Plasma appearance
	Estimation of lipoproteins (qualitative or semiqualitative)
	Special tests (when necessary)
	Post-heparin lipolytic activity
	Ultracentrifugation
	Skin fibroblast culture (for research only)
Primary versus Secondary	Exclude secondary causes
Familial	Screen relatives
Treatment	Diet
	Drugs
	Surgery (rarely)

tal, using NHLBI criteria, only 30% to 35% of the patients who require surgery for atherosclerosis have hyperlipidemia. It is not possible to define an absolute cut-off point for cholesterol or triglyceride values. In our society, levels of these lipids that are considered to be safe are not known. In many African or Asian countries, where the average serum cholesterol is less than 150 mg/100 ml, atherosclerosis is virtually nonexistent. The essential problem for the clinician is to distinguish between a *statistically normal* cholesterol value and a desirable (*optimal*) one, which may be as low as 150 to 200 mg/100 ml. And, in the final analysis, nothing can substitute for the judgment of an individual physician treating individual patients.

Management of Hyperlipidemia and Prevention of Atherosclerosis

Several recent studies have created uncertainty as to whether correction of risk factors will protect the patient from developing atherosclerosis or whether it will reverse atherosclerosis once it has begun. The danger of any particular treatment, whether for hyperlipidemia or for the other predisposing factors, must be balanced against the possible benefits from the treatment.

W. B. Kannel, MD, has summarized one point of view very well:

If he [the physician] elects to proceed on the incomplete evidence available, he can take comfort from the fact that the measures advocated are good health practices and have other health benefits. Who can seriously argue with the general merit of a program that advocates maintenance of lean body weight, a less-rich diet, physical fitness, giving up cigarettes, and control of hypertension, diabetes, and hyperlipidemia?

A number of large-scale dietary intervention programs in the Western countries, aimed at lowering serum cholesterol, have not yielded consistent results. The Coronary Drug Project, a seven-year study, has recently been completed and analyzed. It represented a secondary trial, because the participants, who included only men in the United States, had had one or more myocardial infarctions. Four drugs – dextrothyroxine, conjugated estrogens, clofibrate, and nicotinic acid – were used, all of which lowered serum lipids to varying degrees. The drugs were not very effective in reducing cholesterol levels or in decreasing cardiovascular mortality or overall mortality as compared with the control group receiving the placebo. Estrogen and dextrothyroxine were discontinued because of increased complications reported by patients in the treatment groups. Some of the participants did not have hyperlipidemia. The degree of cholesterol lowering was at best 10% for patients on the most effective regimen – nicotinic acid. Therefore, it is conceivable that more favorable results would have been obtained with younger subjects without coronary disease, preselected for hyperlipidemia, who were given a more potent hypocholesterolemic agent.

The Lipid Research Clinics program of the NHLBI has em-

barked on a primary prevention trial with cholestyramine. Approximately 3,800 randomly selected men are being treated with this drug in a double-blind protocol. The participants selected are free of clinical symptoms associated with coronary disease, but they must have elevated levels of LDL or type II hyperlipidemia. It is hoped that this study will provide definitive information on whether or not lowering cholesterol or LDL levels will protect an individual from atherosclerosis.

In summary, at present the major presumed benefit of lowering serum lipids – reduction in deaths from coronary heart disease – is unproven.

Dietary Recommendations

Apart from the consideration of overt hyperlipidemia, dietary recommendations for the general population of the United States have been proposed by committees of the American Heart Association, the National Academy of Sciences, and the Inter-Society Commission for Heart Disease Resources. These recommendations include achieving and maintaining ideal body weight, reducing the total intake of saturated fat, and decreasing cholesterol intake. Some experts in the area of nutrition also recommend that polyunsaturated fat be substituted for saturated fat.

Diet is the method of treating hyperlipidemia with the least number of side effects. Several therapeutic diets have been prepared by the National Heart, Lung and Blood Institute and by the American Heart Association for patients with hypercholesterolemia and hypertriglyceridemia with the specific hyperlipidemia phenotypes. A diet booklet is only a first step; it is likely to be of only very limited value without the input of a dietitian or physician. Plasma cholesterol and triglyceride levels respond differently to dietary changes. Weight reduction and caloric restriction are quite effective in most patients with hypertriglyceridemia, but they are usually much less effective in lowering serum cholesterol. Plasma cholesterol concentrations, on the other hand, are affected more by the ratio of polyunsaturated to saturated fat in the diet (P/S ratio), and by the total intake of cholesterol, than by weight reduction. The P/S ratio is quantitatively more important than the cholesterol consumption in lowering plasma cholesterol levels.

A high intake of alcohol and of simple sugars may induce endogenous hypertriglyceridemia in some individuals and may exacerbate the condition if it preexists. Endogenous hypertriglyceridemia, due to chylomicronemia, indicates an inability to catabolize dietary triglyceride. It is best controlled by reducing total fat intake, as well as by weight reduction and abstinence from alcohol. Furthermore, there is some evidence that diets rich in polyunsaturates may reduce serum triglyceride as well as cholesterol levels.

The means by which dietary polyunsaturated fats reduce cholesterol levels is unknown. Several mechanisms have been studied, but none has been clearly established. The possibilities include the following: (1) a change in LDL structure, so that it binds and transports less cholesterol; (2) an increased biliary excretion of cholesterol; (3) an increase in LDL catabolism; (4) a decrease in LDL synthesis; or (5) a shift of cholesterol and LDL from the plasma to another body compartment (eg, to the liver).

In the average American diet, the P/S ratio is only about 0.3. For a therapeutic diet to lower plasma cholesterol in a patient with severe type II hyperlipidemia, it is recommended that the ratio be increased to 2. To accomplish this, the patient must consume about four tablespoons of polyunsaturated fats or vegetable oil per day. One of these can be a polyunsaturated margarine, while the other three should be liquid oils, because vegetable oils differ in their content of polyunsaturated fat. For example, safflower oil has the highest P/S ratio, about 9; sunflower seed oil and corn oil have ratios of about 5; soy bean oil, about 3; peanut and olive oil, about 1.5; and cottonseed oil, about 2.

Coconut oil, used to prepare nondairy products, contains plentiful short- to medium-chain fatty acids, which are saturated; it is atherogenic in some animals. Animal fats, particularly organ meats such as kidney, liver, and brains, also contain plentiful saturated fats and cholesterol. Meats with less-saturated fat include fish, poultry, and veal. The more marbled the meat, the higher the content of saturated fat.

The average egg yolk contains approximately 250 to 300 mg of cholesterol. Since the average daily American intake of cholesterol is about 600 mg, two egg yolks can provide nearly all of this. Saturated fat also abounds in such dairy products as butter, whole milk, and cream. A therapeutic diet should include skim milk or low-fat milk as a substitute for whole milk. The Voluntary Labeling Act of the United States Food and Drug Administration has required that manufacturers of

food list the ingredients on the label in the order of their preponderance. Thus, with many margarines, it is possible to determine the type of fat as well as the P/S ratio. The first ingredient listed should be a liquid oil, to attain the highest possible P/S ratio. Usually, a higher P/S ratio is associated with softer margarines.

The dietary treatment of the hyperlipidemias by phenotypes is summarized in Table III. Dietary fat restriction is recommended to control type I hyperlipidemia. Since patients with primary type I are usually children, it is recommended that their diet be supplemented with fat-soluble vitamins as well as with medium-chain triglycerides. For type II, the diet should have a high P/S ratio, and cholesterol should be restricted to less than 300 mg per day. For type IIb, the recommended diet is a combination of that used for types II and IV. Because polyunsaturated fats are as caloric as saturated fats, obese patients should be carefully monitored to help them avoid excessive weight gain. The diets for patients with type IIb or type III hyperlipidemia are virtually the same; with type IV, emphasis is on weight reduction, restriction of alcohol (daily consumption not to exceed 2 oz of whiskey, gin, rum, or vodka, etc; 10 oz of beer; or 5 oz of a dry table wine), and limitation of sweets or free sugars.

Diabetes mellitus and alcoholism are the most frequent secondary causes of type V. The patient with type V typically appears in the emergency room or clinic with severe abdominal pain. Although these attacks can be medically controlled, they can be fatal when associated with acute pancreatitis.

In summary, there are dietary variations for treating exogenous hypertriglyceridemia, endogenous hypertriglyceridemia, and elevated LDL cholesterol. The recommended diets are more complex when more than one of these conditions exists. Also, concomitant occurrence of diabetes mellitus, obesity, hypertension, and congestive heart failure must be taken into account when prescribing a diet for a patient with hyperlipidemia.

Drug Therapy for Hyperlipidemia

There are no precise criteria for drug therapy in the treatment of hyperlipidemia. Important considerations in prescribing medication are the age of the patient; the severity of the hyperlipidemia; the clinical manifestations, including those of arteriosclerosis; the family history; and the presence of coexisting diseases.

The combination of diet and drug therapy is more effective

than drug therapy alone. In providing treatment for the patient, the physician should emphasize that diet and drugs are not curative; however, they can help control hyperlipidemia only as long as the patient complies. There are currently five drugs indicated for the treatment of hyperlipidemia in the United States: clofibrate, cholestyramine, nicotinic acid, dextrothyroxine, and β-sitosterol.

Clofibrate is chlorophenoxyisobutyrate, an ester that is rapidly converted to an acid in the body. It is effective in reducing concentrations of endogenous triglycerides and VLDL in a dosage of 2 gm per day. It can be expected to lower plasma triglyceride concentrations by about 20% to 25%. Experience has shown it to be less effective in lowering cholesterol, with the average reduction about 5% to 10%. The precise mechanism of the action of clofibrate is unknown. It probably has a direct effect on the liver – exerting a major effect on synthesis and/or secretion of hepatic VLDL. In addition, there appears to be a peripheral inhibition of lipolysis in adipose-tissue sites. This results in a decreased release of free fatty acids, which would otherwise be transported to the liver and enhance VLDL synthesis. In addition, there may be a stimulation of adipose-tissue lipoprotein-lipase activity.

The Coronary Drug Project evaluated the beneficial effects of clofibrate administration. Prior to this study, there had been encouraging reports on its use in patients with coronary artery disease and angina pectoris. However, the results from the Drug Project's investigation showed that clofibrate therapy did not protect postcoronary patients from myocardial infarction. Also, there was no reduction in cardiovascular mortality in any subgroup of patients or in the entire group overall. Although clofibrate is usually well tolerated, side effects in patients receiving the medication included gallstones, thrombophlebitis, pulmonary embolism, congestive heart failure, and decreased libido. However, the overall incidence of significant side effects is relatively low.

Cholestyramine is an ion-exchange resin that is not absorbed from the intestine. However, the precise mechanism of its hypocholesterolemic action is unknown. It binds bile acids, increasing their fecal excretion. Cholestyramine lowers cholesterol and LDL levels when the daily dosage is in the range of 16 gm to 24 gm per day. The average reduction is 15% to 20% over and above the effect produced by diet.

The drug causes a net loss of bile acids and, presumably, an increased synthesis of these substances as well as of cholesterol in the liver. In patients with a history of familial hypercholesterolemia, cholestyramine therapy has been reported to increase the fractional catabolic rate of LDL. It may in some way drain the available pool of LDL or LDL-cholesterol. Its major side effects on the gastrointestinal tract are increased fullness, bloating, and constipation. Constipation may be quite severe in a small percentage of patients but can often be controlled by stool softeners.

Nicotinic acid or niacin has been shown to lower concentrations of LDL, VLDL, cholesterol, and triglyceride. It may have a direct effect in blocking lipoprotein synthesis in the liver. It also has a pronounced inhibitory effect on adipose-tissue lipolysis, decreasing the circulating level of fatty acids and decreasing hepatic VLDL synthesis.

Experience has shown that nicotinic acid is more potent than clofibrate in reducing cholesterol levels. The Coronary Drug Project reported that nicotinic acid reduced cholesterol by about 10% and triglycerides by 26%. However, the drug did not reduce overall morbidity or mortality from coronary artery disease as compared with that of the control group. The incidence of nonfatal myocardial infarctions was decreased from about 12% to 9%.

There are potential complications associated with the use of nicotinic acid. Patients may have gastrointestinal symptoms such as nausea and diarrhea. Cutaneous flushing occurs in all patients, but it may be lessened if the drug is taken with meals. Flushing may occur in some patients taking a dose as low as 50 mg to 100 mg. Therefore, it may be necessary to build up gradually to the maximum dose, but in others the maintenance level may be reached within three days, as follows: 250 mg is administered t.i.d. after meals on the first day; 500 mg t.i.d. on the second day; and 1 gm t.i.d. on the third day. Thus, a final dosage of 3 gm per day is obtained. In most patients, the flushing that may occur disappears after two or three days. However, the flushing may recur periodically. Another potential side effect is hepatotoxicity, although it is usually not encountered with 3 gm per day dosage. Nevertheless, liver function tests should be monitored. Finally, this medication may exacerbate hyperuricemia and hyperglycemia. Contraindications for the use of nicotinic acid are diabetes mellitus, active peptic ulcer, hepatic dysfunction, gouty arthritis, and, of course, a patient history of allergic reaction to the medication.

The fourth drug indicated for treatment of hyperlipidemia is sodium dextrothyroxine. This agent is the dextroisomer of the thyroid hormone. Generally, it is more effective in lowering cholesterol than in increasing general metabolic processes. As with the other drugs used for treating hyperlipidemia, the precise mechanism of its action is not known. Thyroid hormones, in general, increase both synthetic and catabolic processes. Triglycerides are slightly reduced, while cholesterol is decreased by about 10%. The usual dosage of the medication is 2 mg to 6 mg per day; this dosage should be attained by increases of 1 mg to 2 mg monthly.

The Coronary Drug Project discontinued the use of sodium dextrothyroxine because of a higher incidence of fatal arrhythmias, new myocardial infarctions, and overall mortality in the group receiving the medication. Its usage is therefore contraindicated in patients with arrhythmia, congestive heart failure, or known coronary artery disease. If the drug is used, it should be restricted to young patients with hypercholesterolemia who do not have coronary artery disease.

β-sitosterol, a plant sterol similar to cholesterol in its structure, is another drug indicated for treating hyperlipidemia. The recommended dose is from 3 gm to 6 gm orally (in suspension form) before meals. The medication lowers LDL cholesterol by approximately 10%, but it does not significantly reduce triglycerides. Diarrhea is the most common side effect.

Other drugs still in the experimental stage or not specifically indicated for treatment of hyperlipidemia are estrogens, progestins, and anabolic steroids. The value of conjugated estrogens was also assessed by the Coronary Drug Project. Although they lowered LDL and increased HDL, they were discontinued because of an increased incidence of intravascular clotting and thromboembolism. Other side effects included testicular softening, breast enlargement and breast tenderness in men. Thus, at this time, estrogens are not recommended for the treatment of hyperlipidemia. Progestins, such as norethindrone acetate, have been used in women with severe type V hyperlipidemia to reduce the hypertriglyceridemia. Their mode of action may be to enhance the activity of lipoprotein lipase in adipose tissue. Estrogens, on the other hand, exacerbate type V by increasing triglycerides and are thus contraindicated. Anabolic steroids such as oxandralone have been used by some investigators to treat hypertriglyceridemia in men with type V hyperlipidemia. They, too, probably increase triglyceride lipase activity in adipose tissue.

Neomycin sulfate is an antibiotic with a hypercholesterolemic effect, which may be due to changes in intestinal mo-

tility or intestinal flora. On the other hand, this effect may result from the antibiotic complexing with bile salts. Oral administration of neomycin sulfate has been used experimentally in conjunction with clofibrate to lower LDL and LDL-cholesterol levels in patients with type II hyperlipidemia. The most serious and significant side effects of neomycin sulfate are gastrointestinal discomfort, ototoxicity, and renal toxicity.

Para-aminosalicylic acid is an agent used to treat tuberculosis. It, too, lowers LDL and LDL-cholesterol by 15% to 20%. The most commonly observed side effects are nausea, diarrhea, and abdominal pain.

A number of agents similar to clofibrate have been produced. One of these is halofenate, which lowers uric acid as well as triglyceride levels. However, gastrointestinal hemorrhage has been associated with its use. Tibric acid has been found to lower both cholesterol and triglycerides and is reportedly more potent than clofibrate. Probucol decreases cholesterol absorption and lowers plasma cholesterol by 10% to 20%, but it has no significant effect on plasma triglyceride. In experimental studies, dietary pectin and an unknown substance that is present in soybean protein have been noted to have hypocholesterolemic actions.

It may be that a combination of agents that affect different steps in lipoprotein and lipid synthesis or catabolism will be required to achieve optimal lowering of lipids. However, if an agent is to be acceptable, it must not interfere with cell division, growth, or maturation.

An entirely different approach is to develop drugs that are not necessarily hypolipidemic, but that interfere with or reverse cholesterol deposition in the arterial wall. If one assumes that HDL is a physiological scavenger of cholesterol, then an agent that could raise HDL without causing untoward side effects would be valuable in preventing atherosclerosis. Conceivably, synthetic agents could be developed that would mimic the structure of plasma lipoproteins and, therefore, interfere with cholesterol deposition.

HYPERTENSION

Hypertension is another of the three major risk factors of premature coronary artery disease. It is the most important single risk factor for cerebrovascular disease, and particularly for cerebral hemorrhage. In physiologic terms, hypertension is often associated with an increased total peripheral resistance and with various changes in cardiac output and total vascular volume. In the early stages of hypertension, an increase in cardiac output may be the primary effect. With chronic hypertension, increased peripheral resistance may predominate. Thus, hypertension may occur whenever there is an imbalance in cardiac output, volume of the vascular tree, and vascular resistance.

The nervous system and the endocrine-renal system are of major importance in the etiology and persistence of a hypertensive state. Both the central and peripheral nervous systems are involved in the regulation of resistance in the vascular bed, which is mediated in large part through the contractile state of arteriolar smooth muscle. Neurogenic regulation of blood pressure is also brought into play through baroreceptors located in the carotid body, the aortic arch, probably in the midbrain, and possibly through peripheral nerves in the renal cortex. The endocrine-renal system involves a series of intricate interactions, largely between the kidney and adrenal cortex. These are partially mediated by renin, angiotensin, and aldosterone, and influence sodium and potassium retention. The neurogenic and endocrine-renal systems are themselves interrelated; for example, there is some evidence that renin can affect vasomotor tone by actions on the midbrain.

Definitions of hypertension vary with the age of the patient. For infants, a value of 90/60 is suggested; preteenage children, 120/80; teenagers, 130/80; and in adults, 140/90. It is my opinion that an adult with a blood pressure value of 140/90 should be carefully monitored. Treatment should be provided for the patient if the value persists above this level. According to life insurance statistics, there is a stepwise increase in mortality for each increase in blood pressure. The younger the patient when high blood pressure develops, the more serious is the prognosis. The incidence of hypertension in the United States has been called "alarming," and statistics provided by the American Heart Association indicate that it is adequately treated in perhaps only one out of eight patients.

The estimated number of American adults affected by hypertension is 23 to 25 million, according to the AHA; of

Table VIII.
Workup of a patient to establish the presence of hypertension.

Urinalysis (urine culture when sediment is abnormal)
Serum creatinine
Creatinine clearance
Serum electrolytes
ECG
Four-hour urine collection for VMA
Rapid-sequence intravenous pyelogram
Plasma renin concentration
(Chest x-ray when indicated)

For Suspected Cases

Renovascular hypertension	Selective renal arteriogram
	Renal vein renin concentrations
Primary hyperaldosteronism	Plasma renin concentration
	Plasma aldosterone
	Observe effect of high-salt diet
Pheochromocytoma	Urinary catecholamines
	Regitine or tyramine test

these, one half are undetected, one fourth are being treated, and only one half of these are treated adequately. These statistics point to a deplorable health situation. Fortunately, the most recently available statistics suggest that the situation is improving because of better detection and treatment.

One of the controversies among physicians concerning the evaluation of hypertension is the extent to which a workup should be pursued (Table VIII). A majority of patients with hypertension (as many as 85% to 90%) have essential hypertension, and a diagnostic evaluation to identify a secondary cause is usually negative. A recently published estimate of the cost for detecting secondary hypertension was approximately $2,000 per patient; this also was the amount for evaluation of a patient with renovascular hypertension. Using this figure, the projected cost of screening the entire population of the United States would be the staggering figure of $10 to $13 billion.

Since adequate and relatively safe treatment is available, it becomes even more urgent to screen and treat patients with hypertension. Education of the public is essential. People should be aware that (1) they should have their blood pressure checked, and (2) after hypertension has been detected, therapy should be initiated and continued. Obviously, if a patient is identified as having a curable form of hypertension, it is preferable to remove the cause rather than subject him to a lifetime of treatment.

The most frequently encountered curable forms of hypertension are (1) renal artery stenosis of atherosclerotic and nonatherosclerotic origin; (2) dysfunction of the adrenal gland, including aldosterone-secreting adenomas, Cushing's disease, and pheochromocytomas; (3) unilateral chronic renal parenchymal disease, such as nephrosclerosis and pyelonephritis; (4) coarctation of the aorta; and (5) hypertension caused by the use of oral contraceptives. Other curable forms less frequently seen include increased intracranial pressure, hyperthyroidism and hypothyroidism, polycythemia, burns, eclampsia, and arteriovenous fistula. Certain of these conditions are associated with high cardiac output, eg, hyperthyroidism and arteriovenous fistula. Again, it is emphasized that these curable forms comprise only 10% to 15% of the total population that has hypertension.

Diagnosis

General: An initial workup of the patient should include (1) a measure of the serum electrolytes, BUN, and creatinine; (2) urinalysis, including renal sediment; (3) electrocardiogram; (4) intravenous pyelogram (IVP), concentrating on the first 30 to 60 seconds of uptake of the dye; and (5) chest x-ray. If the findings of all these tests are negative, the physician should proceed with treatment, carefully assessing the patient's response to therapy. If the patient does not respond or if there are unusual features, such as the development of hypokalemia with cyclic or periodic hypertension, further diagnostic study is warranted.

Drug-induced hypertension: Laboratory tests are not always necessary for diagnosis. For example, in young women taking oral contraceptives, it may be worthwhile to discontinue the medication to determine if blood pressure will normalize. Other drugs that may cause hypertension include the sympathetic amines, cocaine, and amphetamines. The monoamine oxidase inhibitors, in conjunction with tyramine or sympathetic amines, also may induce severe hypertension.

Renovascular hypertension: This form may be a result of parenchymal or vascular disease of the kidney but, paradoxically, hypertension may cause renal disease. For example, prolonged hypertension may lead to pathological changes in the kidney known as nephrosclerosis. In the accelerated form of hypertension, renal insufficiency is a prominent finding. Renovascular hypertension may be caused by disease affecting one or both kidneys. Most commonly, there is partial blockage of one or both of the renal arteries from an atherosclerotic plaque, or from a condition known as *fibromuscular hyperplasia.* When the latter occurs in the presence of hypertension, it is more ominous than in normotensive patients, because it is more likely to be progressive.

Corrective surgery may or may not be curative in renal artery stenosis. Follow-up angiographic studies are necessary to determine whether the disease has progressed. When the obstruction is severe enough to reduce blood flow to the kidneys by more than 50%, the kidney with the decreased blood flow responds by releasing a proteolytic enzyme called *renin* from the juxtaglomerular apparatus of the renal afferent arteriole (Figure 9). The renin level is increased in the renal vein of the affected kidney. This hormone, in turn, causes the conversion of a renin substrate (made in the liver) to angiotensin I, a decapeptide. Angiotensin I is then acted on by a pulmonary factor called *converting enzyme* to form angiotensin II, an octapeptide. Angiotensin II causes constriction of arterioles and stimulates the zona glomerulosa of the adrenal cortex to increase aldosterone secretion. Some evidence from experimental animals indicates that angiotensin may affect the vasomotor tone of arterioles by influencing baroreceptors and mechanical receptors in the midbrain.

An IVP, frequently part of a routine workup, detects approximately 70% of renovascular hypertension. To pinpoint the site of the lesion, an arteriogram is required. To determine if a unilateral lesion reduces renal blood flow to the point of requiring surgery, it is necessary to measure the concentration of plasma renin. (The concentration of this substance may be altered in patients on a salt-restriction diet or by the use of diuretics.) Surgery should be recommended only if there is hypersecretion of renin by the affected kidney and a suppression of renin excretion by the unaffected kidney.

The renin and aldosterone functions are interrelated. The renin-angiotensin relationship is the major one involved in regulating aldosterone secretion (Figure 9). However, an increase in the concentration of serum potassium and, to a lesser extent, ACTH can also stimulate aldosterone release. Primary hyperaldosteronism, or Conn's syndrome, refers to the overproduction of aldosterone, usually by a single adenoma of the adrenal cortex. This overproduction leads to (1) suppression of renin release by the kidney, (2) sodium and water reabsorption in the distal convoluted tubules of the kidney, and (3) potassium loss. Plasma volume expands, renal per-

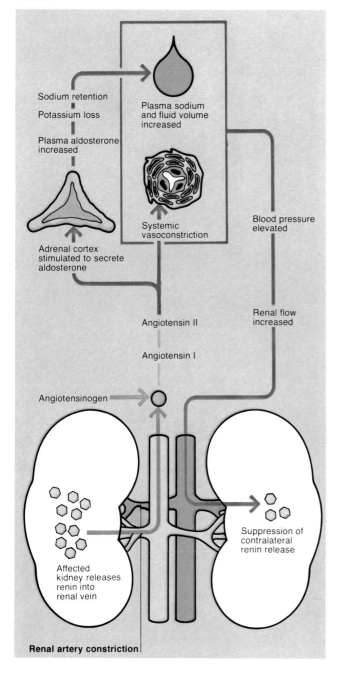

Figure 9. Pathway of abnormal function of kidney having reduced blood flow due to blockage of renal arteries.

Sodium retention

Potassium loss

Plasma aldosterone increased

Plasma sodium and fluid volume increased

Adrenal cortex stimulated to secrete aldosterone

Systemic vasoconstriction

Blood pressure elevated

Angiotensin II

Renal flow increased

Angiotensin I

Angiotensinogen

Suppression of contralateral renin release

Affected kidney releases renin into renal vein

Renal artery constriction

fusion is increased, and renin secretion is suppressed. Thus, in primary hyperaldosteronism the concentration of renin is low and aldosterone concentration is high. If these measurements are not available, an alternate diagnostic test is the administration of spironolactone, a specific aldosterone antagonist. If administration of this substance corrects the blood pressure elevation as well as the hypokalemia within two or three weeks, it suggests a diagnosis of primary hyperaldosteronism. Also, a high sodium intake probably will produce hypokalemia in these patients. Other findings that suggest this diagnosis are the occurrence of hypokalemia after the first few weeks of treatment with a mild thiazide diuretic and loss of serum potassium greater than 30 mg per 24 hours.

Periodic episodic hypertension: The occurrence of periodic episodic hypertension, pounding headaches, and elevated blood sugar suggests pheochromocytoma, a tumor of the adrenal medulla. In about one half of the cases of pheochromocytoma, the hypertension is sustained rather than episodic. Diagnosis may be established by 24-hour urine collections for the measurement of catecholamines (ephinephrine and norepinephrine) and their metabolites (vanillylmandelic acid and metanephrine). If the patient has a hypertensive crisis, adrenergic blocking agents (eg, phentolamine and phenoxybenzamine) can correct the elevated blood pressure. It may be diagnostically useful to collect urine four hours after the crisis.

Cushing's syndrome: Another adrenal-related cause of hypertension is Cushing's syndrome, in which there is an overproduction of adrenocortical steroids. If this diagnosis is suspected – and usually there are other clinical features in addition to hypertension which may suggest it – then measurements of plasma cortisol are in order. Cushing's disease interferes with a person's normal circadian rhythm for cortisol secretion. Therefore, measurements of the fasting, basal level of cortisol and 4 PM cortisol should be performed. There is also a loss of cortisol secretion regulation, which is tested by dexamethasone administration.

Renin measurements in hypertension: As previously noted, renin release may be excessive in a patient with an ischemic kidney and low in the presence of primary hyperaldosteronism (Figure 9). J. H. Laragh, MD, has suggested the utility of renin measurements in the classification and prognosis of hypertension.

Laragh postulated that patients with low or normal renin secretion are less likely to develop cardiovascular sequelae than are individuals with high renin-secretion levels. The proposed mechanism of the hypertension in patients with low renin is that the arterial bed has a volume overload; the treatment consists of using diuretics. Patients with high concentrations of plasma renin are thought to have a disproportionate increase in peripheral vascular resistance; the recommended treatment for these patients is a β-adrenergic blocking agent, such as propranolol. Actually, the use of propranolol for treating all varieties of essential hypertension is becoming more widespread. The volume type of hypertension may be converted to the vasoconstrictor type of sodium depletion. A provocative test to stimulate renin secretion may be carried out by administering the diuretic furosemide to a patient who is on an unrestricted diet and is kept ambulant for five hours. Under these conditions, the normal patient response (determined by serum analysis) is an increase in renin excretion that results from the reduction in effective blood volume; patients may then be separated into categories of low renin, normal renin, and high renin secretion.

Treatment of Hypertension

Since both obesity and excessive salt consumption exacerbate hypertension, modification of diet is an important aspect of treatment. Unfortunately, weight reduction per se is not usually sufficient to control blood pressure except for obese patients with mild hypertension. Salt restriction is an effective measure in controlling hypertension. However, if drug therapy is not prescribed, the patient's salt intake should be limited to 500 mg or less per day. But it is difficult to get most patients to limit their salt intake to this extent. If diuretics are used in conjunction with salt restriction, the patient's salt intake may be increased to about 3 gm per day. For mild cases of hypertension, mild sedatives and rest may also help. However, for moderate or severe hypertension, other measures should be used.

A variety of drugs are available for treatment of hypertension. A detailed discussion of these agents is beyond the scope of this review, but oral diuretic agents usually are the first and most frequently employed medications. They decrease blood pressure, do not lead to patient tolerance, tend to increase the effectiveness of other antihypertensive drugs, and have a relatively low incidence of side effects.

Oral diuretics: The most frequently used diuretic agents are the thiazides. Skin rashes, hyperuricemia, hyperglycemia, renal toxicity, and hypokalemia are possible side effects. Some patients may require potassium supplementation. Other diuretic agents, such as spironolactone and triamterene, do not cause potassium loss, but they are less potent than the thiazide diuretics. Spironolactone is an aldosterone antagonist especially effective in the treatment of primary hyperaldosteronism and possibly in low-renin hypertension as well. It may cause breast enlargement and tenderness in some male patients, which, in rare instances, may persist.

For patients with repeated diastolic blood pressure measurements between 90 and 110 mm Hg, oral diuretics should be tried first. If these are not effective, or if the diastolic blood pressure is between 110 and 130, an additional agent, eg, methyldopa, a rauwolfia analog, or propranolol, may be required. Alternatively, a more potent diuretic such as furosemide may be prescribed.

Combination therapy: Combination drug therapy may be indicated in some patients to decrease the total dosage of an individual drug. For example, if an oral diuretic is prescribed in conjunction with either methyldopa or rauwolfia, a third drug, such as hydralazine, may be added if necessary. The general approach should be as follows: begin with an oral diuretic; if satisfactory blood-pressure reduction is not obtained after two or three weeks, add methyldopa, rauwolfia, propranolol, or substitute the more potent furosemide for the original diuretic agent. After one month, if further reduction in blood pressure is required, various combinations of these agents may be used or hydralazine may be added.

Rauwolfia: The rauwolfia drugs are alkaloids that cause depletion of norepinephrine and epinephrine from sympathetic nerve endings. They decrease peripheral vascular resistance, slow the pulse, and lower the blood pressure. Maximum effectiveness is usually achieved after two to three weeks of therapy. The most serious side effect of these drugs is depression, which may cause suicidal tendencies in some patients. Exacerbation of peptic ulcers, nasal stuffiness, drowsiness, and impotence also may occur.

Methyldopa: Although the precise mode of methyldopa's action is not understood, it is known to inhibit the decarboxylation of dopa to dopamine in the norepinephrine synthesis pathway. It has not, however, been established that the decarboxylase inhibition is responsible for the antihypertensive property of methyldopa. Tissue levels of norepinephrine and epinephrine are reduced by this drug, possibly due to the displacement of norepinephrine from adrenergic nerve endings by a metabolite of methyldopa, α-methyl-norepinephrine. Finally, methyldopa also decreases CNS sympathetic control over vasoconstriction. The net effect of this drug's actions, then, is to decrease peripheral resistance in the arteriolar bed. Methyldopa is an effective agent even in the presence of impaired renal function. Side effects are relatively few, the most common being lassitude and, less commonly, hemolytic anemia. Liver dysfunction and a positive Coombs' test may also occur. The drug is usually started at 250 mg, two or three times daily; larger doses may be given if necessary, provided the smaller dose is tolerated.

Hydralazine: Hydralazine is useful in combination with other drugs, but not as a sole agent. Its mode of action probably involves effects on peripheral arterioles. It has a stimulatory effect on the heart, increasing cardiac output. However, it may exacerbate angina pectoris, and it must be used with caution in patients with clinically symptomatic coronary artery disease. Tolerance to hydralazine may develop in some patients. The starting dose is 10 mg to 25 mg q.i.d.; the dosage may then be increased at weekly intervals. The most serious side effect is the development of a syndrome resembling lupus erythematosus, which usually is reversible.

Guanethidine: In addition to the above agents, guanethidine, a ganglion-blocking agent with sympatholytic action, can be used in conjunction with oral diuretic agents and with methyldopa or hydralazine for treating severe hypertension. The starting dosage is generally 25 mg daily, in one or two divided doses. The dosage may be increased at one- to two-week intervals. Side effects include diarrhea, failure to ejaculate, and orthostatic hypotension. The last is the most serious, but it may be avoided by carefully titrating the amount of medication. Also, the addition of an oral diuretic to the patient's therapy will lessen the likelihood of orthostatic hypotension by decreasing the required dosage of guanethidine.

Propranolol; clonidine: The use of propranolol in the treatment of hypertension has been mentioned. It blocks beta-adrenergic receptors and, according to Laragh, is particularly useful for hypertensive patients who have high renin levels. Clonidine, another agent, acts primarily on the central nervous system and is useful in treating patients with orthostatic hypotension. For the acute hypertensive crisis, diazoxide, nitroprusside, and guanethidine are the drugs of choice, whereas phentolamine is important in relieving the hypertensive emergency associated with a pheochromocytoma.

Smoking

Smoking is the third major risk factor in coronary artery disease, and numerous clinical reports describe an association between smoking and peripheral atherosclerosis. It further increases the risk in patients with hypertension and hyperlipidemia. Younger patients who smoke have an increased risk by twofold to threefold for developing clinical coronary artery disease. Its effect is independent of other risk factors such as hypercholesterolemia and hypertension, although smoking may exacerbate the actions of other risk factors on coronary artery disease.

Obviously, smokers who inhale suffer greater risk than those who do not. Although some investigators have claimed that smoking cigars or a pipe has fewer associated risks than smoking cigarettes, this remains to be assessed further.

When nicotine is administered in very high doses to animals, it can produce calcification and necrosis of the arterial media, a condition that is similar to the nonobstructing lesion of Mönckeberg's arteriosclerosis. However, in these studies, nicotine has not been observed to cause atherosclerosis. Some investigators have postulated that carbon monoxide and an increased concentration of carboxyhemoglobin in the blood are responsible for the increased risk of atherosclerotic complications in the smoker. They have suggested that (1) decreasing the oxygen supply available to peripheral tissues might be of particular importance in peripheral arteriosclerosis, and (2) carboxyhemoglobin levels may go as high as 20% in smokers who inhale cigarettes. Persons who smoke low-nicotine and low-tar cigarettes may be protected more from lung cancer than from coronary artery disease, because their exposure to carbon monoxide is not as effectively reduced.

A common result of giving up smoking is substantial weight gain (possibly as much as 20 to 25 lb). Therefore, patients who also want to lose weight should establish a diet before attempting to give up smoking.

Secondary Risk Factors

PHYSICAL INACTIVITY

Exercise results in caloric expenditure and thus helps to determine whether an individual maintains or loses weight. Theoretically, if caloric intake remains constant and caloric output is increased through exercise, weight loss should occur. However, dietary management is usually required as well, since exercise alone may increase appetite.

Exercise increases the amount of oxygen carried to and extracted by the tissues, thus increasing the pulse and respiration rates. The better the individual's physical condition, the slower the pulse rate needed to satisfy the increased oxygen requirement. The term "aerobic capacity" is defined as the maximum oxygen uptake that can be sustained during exercise. Various cardiovascular diseases, as well as senility, cause a decrease in aerobic capacity.

Many studies have described the protective effect of physical activity. Some investigators have claimed that vigorous physical activity protects an individual from coronary artery disease. Others have challenged this interpretation. In many studies, the groups were not involved with vigorous physical activity, eg, the London Bus Driver vs Conductor Study. The Framingham Study observed a relationship between coronary artery disease and lack of fitness. However, physical activity was inferred from vital capacity, weight gain, and resting pulse rate, and was not directly measured. At least one of these parameters, the vital capacity, is not correlated with physical activity, nor is weight gain necessarily correlated. However, individuals who scored poorly on all three parameters had approximately a fivefold increase in mortality.

In summary, evidence suggests that physical exercise may protect individuals from coronary artery disease, but the findings are not scientifically conclusive. The position has been well stated by the Committee on Exercise of the American Heart Association: "...we do not consider it justifiable to advocate widespread adoption of vigorous exercise programs purely on the ground that exercise alone will prevent heart disease." Several benefits, however, are derived from exercise programs, such as improvement of general health and well-being, and increased work capacity. These are very useful adjuncts for patients recovering from myocardial infarctions, cardiovascular surgery, cerebrovascular accidents, and other illnesses. Exercise may also be helpful in controlling obesity, hypertension, or hyperlipidemia. Undoubtedly, exercise is the most important single ingredient in a rehabilitation program. It must be individualized for the patient, and may vary in the degree of physical effort required. A cardiac patient's personal physician is best qualified to prescribe the precise exercise program.

DIABETES MELLITUS

A previous Scope monograph has provided a detailed review of diabetes mellitus; thus, this discussion is limited to the relationship between diabetes and atherosclerotic complications. There is little doubt that there is an increased incidence of coronary artery disease in patients with diabetes mellitus. Vascular diseases are very common in diabetic patients and account for about three quarters of their deaths. Over one half of these deaths are caused by coronary atherosclerosis, followed by cerebral and then renal arteriosclerotic complications. It is estimated that there are at least 10 million patients with diabetes in the United States, most of whom are over the age of 40. Because of the relationship between hyperlipidemia and atherosclerosis, it is important to monitor cholesterol and triglyceride measurements in these patients. As previously discussed, diabetes is one of the most common causes of secondary hyperlipidemia.

The patient with diabetes is particularly susceptible to peripheral vascular disease of the lower extremities. The large vessels of the extremities may be affected by occlusive atherosclerotic lesions, which are virtually indistinguishable from those occurring in patients without diabetes. Also, calcification of the large vessels (Mönckeberg's sclerosis) may develop. When this syndrome is present, calcification occurs in the smooth-muscle cells present in the media of the large-sized and medium-sized arteries. Patients with diabetes frequently experience the following complications: (1) occlusion of more than one major vessel in the lower extremities, (2) a greater incidence of calcification of the arteries, and (3) an occluded popliteal artery without collateral circulation. Lesions with deposits of hyaline material may be present in smaller arteries and arterioles. Intermittent claudication, pain that occurs during rest, ulcers, and gangrene are signs and symptoms of progressively more severe peripheral arteriosclerosis. In addition to arteriosclerotic changes affecting the extremities, a patient may develop neuropathy with decreased sensation and vibration modalities and an absence of deep tendon reflexes. Finally, patients with diabetes may develop microangiopathy, a lesion characterized by thickening of the basement membranes of capillaries.

Patients with compromised circulation of the extremities

have an increased susceptibility to infection. Fungal infections may lead to gangrene, most commonly caused by *Clostridium perfringens* or *Micrococcus pyogenes*. Gangrene occurs three to five times more frequently in patients with diabetes than in those who are not affected. Surgery may be required, including arterial reconstruction, sympathectomy, and even amputation. The major preventive measures are adequate management of diabetes, correction of risk factors, and proper care of the lower extremities.

Patients with diabetes have an increased incidence of myocardial infarction, and their recovery or survival from infarctions is lower than that reported for patients without diabetes. Thus far, it has not been scientifically proven that careful regulation of blood glucose protects the patient with diabetes from coronary artery disease. However, diabetes is definitely a risk factor, and all risk factors should be vigorously controlled. The American Diabetes Association recently stated that there is now sufficient evidence to conclude that tighter control of blood sugar is likely to reduce vascular complications in diabetics. There is not a consensus of agreement, however, among physicians as to whether this view is correct. The physician must evaluate the patient as to which course of treatment has fewest complications, ie, controlling blood sugar with or without medication versus risking an attack of hypoglycemia. While it is more convenient for the diabetic patient to administer the required amount of insulin in one or two daily doses, this does subject the patient to relatively large variations in blood sugar levels. For most patients, particularly children, it is not practical to recommend multiple daily injections. Various mechanical devices are now being studied which might act as "glucose sensors" and administer a steady quantity of insulin in response to the body's demand for the hormone.

Other areas of investigation which are promising, but in the experimental stage, include transplanting pancreatic islets. Another exciting development was the report of recent studies of a polyol substance, inositol, which was administered to rats with diabetes, and prevented the development of neurological lesions.

For patients with diabetes, it may well be that small-vessel disease affecting the eye, the kidney, and the extremities has a different etiology than large-vessel disease that causes coronary atherosclerosis. In the southwestern United States, there is a group of Indians with a high incidence of diabetes mellitus, obesity, and hypertension. Plasma cholesterol levels are extremely low and there is very little coronary artery disease or death from myocardial infarction. Possibly because of low cholesterol levels, the Indians are protected from large-vessel disease. Nevertheless, they suffer the typical symptoms associated with diabetic small-vessel disease, such as microangiopathy of the eye, kidney, and nerves.

As a general rule, the complications associated with diabetes do not occur until 15 to 20 years after the onset of elevated blood sugar. Until we have the means for more physiologic control of blood sugar in patients with diabetes, it is doubtful if we can determine whether hyperglycemia per se is damaging to patients.

PERSONALITY TYPE AND STRESS

Rosenman, Friedman, and others have popularized the relationship between type A behavior and coronary artery disease; they believe that the central nervous system has an important role in the etiology. The characteristics of the type A personality include consciousness of time, conscientiousness, high standards and principles, critical nature, adherence to the work ethic, and inner-directedness. This contrasts with the type B personality, who is more relaxed, less time-conscious, and is considered to be less prone to heart disease.

An eight-year Western collaborative study, published in 1975 by Rosenman et al, indicated that personality type significantly affects the incidence of coronary artery disease, apart from other risk factors. Several epidemiologists have questioned the methodology and conclusions of the Western collaborative study. Friedman and Rosenman have claimed there is an association between type A behavior, hyperlipidemia, and norepinephrine release in response to stress. The association with hyperlipidemia is not well established. These investigators established the individual's behavior type by personal interview. Other investigators have employed a self-administered test, which may show a weaker correlation with coronary artery disease than the interview. The significance of personality type as a risk factor requires further study.

The stress factor is distinct from personality type. Certain individuals may be more prone to physical and emotional stress, which can exacerbate hypertension or precipitate angina pectoris in susceptible patients with underlying coronary artery disease. In some instances, physicians recommend that patients with coronary disease or myocardial infarction lessen the amount of stress they experience on a day-to-day basis. This recommendation is based on the hypothesis that overactivity of the adrenergic nervous system may exert a deleterious effect on the heart and arteries over a period of time.

OBESITY

Obesity is a very common problem in our society, aggravating several other risk factors, particularly hypertension, hypertriglyceridemia, and diabetes mellitus. Analysis of mortality statistics from insurance data supports the importance of obesity as a risk factor. The Framingham Study established a strong relationship between increased weight gain, angina pectoris, myocardial infarction, and sudden death, and found the correlations more significant for men than for women. However, obesity per se did not correlate well with these findings. Many other epidemiologic studies have not shown a strong association between obesity and coronary artery disease. Autopsy studies have also failed to establish a positive correlation between obesity and the severity of coronary atherosclerosis.

Some investigators have classified obesity as (1) hyperplastic, where there is an increase in the *number* of cells, and (2) hypertrophic, where the *size* of the cell increases. In animal experiments, it is possible to increase the number of adipose-tissue cells by overfeeding early in life. Most adult obesity represents an increase in the size rather than in the number of cells. It has not been established whether or not it is possible to prevent obesity by not overfeeding children.

The only safe way to lose weight is to lower the caloric intake below the amount of energy expended. Crash diets are not recommended. Neither are the high-fat and zero-carbohydrate diets recommended, as they can be dangerous to some patients. It is preferable to have a person change his or her eating habits and adopt a maintenance diet once the desired weight is reached. A loss of 2 lb per week is perfectly adequate for most obese patients. A calorie-restricted, balanced diet in which 45% of the calories come from carbohydrate, 35% from fat, and 20% from protein will allow most patients to lose weight.

DIET AND PREVENTION OF ATHEROSCLEROSIS: SATURATED FAT VS SUGAR

Because of the limited number of adequate autopsy studies, it is very difficult to estimate the death rate from coronary artery disease prior to World War II. There is no question, however, that there was a very substantial decrease in deaths from coronary artery disease in Holland and Norway during World War II, when there was a marked reduction in saturated fat consumption. Also, the American diet contains approximately three times more saturated fat than does the Japanese diet, and the Japanese have a much lower death rate from coronary artery disease than Americans do, although their rate is increasing.

Yudkin and others have attempted to establish a correlation between sugar consumption and coronary artery disease, but the correlation with saturated fat appears more convincing, and the sugar hypothesis remains unproven. For instance, in countries such as Cuba, where the population consumes large amounts of sugar, the mortality from coronary artery disease is low. In other countries where the population has a serum cholesterol level less than 150 mg/100 ml, coronary artery disease is also extremely rare. Although fatty streaks do develop in children, teenagers, and young adults, they do not progress to raised, complicated lesions. In our society, similar fatty streaks develop in most individuals, but it is unclear whether these streaks are precursors of more advanced lesions.

It is not now known whether or not coronary artery disease could be significantly reduced in the United States if diets were modified to lower serum cholesterol levels below 150 mg/100 ml. Dietary measures necessary to achieve such levels would be severe. They would involve changing to a diet consisting largely of grain and wheat products, legumes, nuts, and fruit. Animal fats would be consumed only in very limited quantities, and saturated fat consumption would be markedly diminished. Eggs would be eliminated, with skim milk and cheese made from skim milk constituting the main dairy products. The percentage of calories from carbohydrates would be quite high. Such a rigorous, large-scale dietary program is clearly not practical in the United States today.

It is gratifying to conclude this section on risk factors for atherosclerosis with an encouraging note. Based on the latest data from the National Center for Health Statistics, there has been a very significant reduction in the mortality rate from coronary artery disease in the United States since

1968 (Table IX). The decrease in mortality has been observed in both men and women, regardless of race. As no single factor has been identified to account for the decline, the availability of coronary care units or of coronary bypass surgery cannot be considered a primary contributing factor. It is my opinion that greater public education about risk factors, emphasis on exercise, the importance of dietary management, lowering cholesterol levels, and detection and treatment of hypertension are all contributing factors. Further study will enable us to devise the most effective and practical means of protecting ourselves and our patients from the ravages of atherosclerosis.

SUMMARY

There are three major factors that increase a person's risk for developing premature coronary artery disease: (1) hypercholesterolemia, (2) hypertension, and (3) cigarette smoking. Several secondary risk factors also have been identified, including elevated serum triglycerides, diabetes mellitus, obesity, lack of physical activity, stress, and a tense, over-conscientious personality. There is now evidence that treating severe blood pressure elevations can reduce death from accelerated hypertension, cerebrovascular accidents, renal failure, and hypertensive heart failure. Conclusive scientific proof is not available which suggests that treating risk factors can prevent death from coronary artery disease or affect overall mortality. Several studies now being sponsored by the National Heart, Lung and Blood Institute may clarify the efficacy of current measures used for treating major risk factors. Until better information is available, it seems prudent to intervene when overt risk factors such as hyperlipidemia, hypertension, diabetes, obesity, physical inactivity, and cigarette smoking are identified.

ACKNOWLEDGMENT

The following figure has been reproduced by permission of the authors and publisher.

Figure 2A. Hamilton RL, Havel RJ, Kane JP, et al: Cholestasis: Lamellar structure of the abnormal human serum lipoprotein. *Science* 172: 475-478, 30 Apr 1971. Copyright 1971 by the American Association for the Advancement of Science.

Table IX.
Percent change in death rates from heart attacks in the United States from 1968-1974.

Age Group	White		Nonwhite	
	Men	Women	Men	Women
35-44	−20.6	−20.1	−30.7	−36.8
45-54	−13.6	−14.4	−15.7	−22.4
55-64	−14.6	−15.0	−17.9	−26.3
65-74	−14.4	−20.3	−25.7	−30.3

SECTION II

The Pathogenesis of Human Atherosclerosis

Abel Lazzarini Robertson, Jr., MD, PhD

Professor of Pathology
and
Director
Interdisciplinary Cardiovascular Research
Case Western Reserve University
School of Medicine
Cleveland, Ohio 44106

Nomenclature and Definitions

Arteriosclerosis, atheroma, and *atherosclerosis* are terms often used interchangeably in the medical literature, in spite of their different origins and pathological meaning. The term *arteriosclerosis* was first used by Lobstein in 1829 as a generic anatomicopathological description of several arterial diseases involving degeneration, thickening, and induration of one or more layers of the vascular wall. The term should be used to describe atherosclerosis (a predominantly intimal disease and by far the most common and clinically significant lesion of large- and medium-sized arteries) as well as a variety of other pathological changes affecting the arterial wall.

As shown in Table I, arbitrary subdivisions of arteriosclerosis may be made, based on which arterial layer is most involved in the early stages of disease. It should be emphasized, however, that as the lesions become more severe, there is considerable overlapping of histological changes often masked by unrelated arterial disease.

According to Paré (1575), the word *atheroma* was first used in ancient Greece to describe any "cystic space containing gruel-like material or porridge." Von Haller (1755) used this term to identify arterial lesions containing elevations or plaques with central necrosis and pultaceous content. Marchand (1904) was first to suggest that "fatty" intimal lesions should be considered atheroma rather than arteriosclerosis. He further confused the nomenclature by coining the term *scleroatherosis* to describe lesions in any arterial layer containing abundant lipids.

Virchow (1862) emphasized the presence of inflammatory cells surrounding the atheromatous plaque. He called these lesions *endarteritis chronica sine nodosa.* Councilman (1891) proposed the term *nodular arteriosclerosis* in order to stress the patchy distribution of the lesions. Some authors, such as Pickering (1963), still prefer this nomenclature to all others.

In an attempt to avoid further confusion, the designation *atheroarteriosclerosis* was proposed to define arteriosclerotic lesions. These lesions were characterized by initial involvement of the intima and, to a lesser extent, of the inner media, containing intracellular and extracellular lipids with varying degrees of ground substance involvement, particularly glycosaminoglycans and collagen deposits. Since both fatty and fibroelastic lesions may occur simultaneously or independently in man, this term has had considerably more anatomicopathological meaning than those previously proposed.

In assuming that atheroarteriosclerosis is the most frequent underlying cause of cerebral and coronary artery occlusion, it should be considered an important predisposing factor in cerebral ischemia and myocardial infarction. These are the two most prevalent causes of death due to arterial disease. In this monograph the term *atherosclerosis,* now most commonly used in current medical literature, is used to describe such lesions.

However, it is important to emphasize that atherosclerosis is often used not only to describe the characteristic arterial lesions of this disease but also the accompanying symptoms resulting from secondary ischemia and necrosis of vital organs. This generic use of the term is often inaccurate and confusing. Although atheromatous lesions are exceedingly common in the middle-aged population of developed countries, the arteriopathy often does not progress to the stage where clinical symptoms are induced. In some patients it may remain undetected for many years. As with other metabolic disorders, including diabetes mellitus, atherosclerosis may thus be considered a pathological state or disease of the arterial wall, with subclinical and clinical or symptomatic phases.

The distinction is important because current epidemiological and experimental studies suggest that therapeutic approaches may differ and that the anticipated benefits may be related to the stage of the disease at which treatment is initiated.

Table I.
Classification of the most common types of arteriosclerosis.

Name	Predominant initial lesion	Arterial size
Atherosclerosis	Intima (inner media)	Large and medium arteries
Mönckeberg's arteriosclerosis	Media	Large and medium arteries
Arteriolar sclerosis	Intima/media	Arterioles

Other arterial lesions that may accompany arteriosclerosis

Name	Predominant initial lesion	Arterial size
Endoarteritis obliterans	Intima	Small arteries and arterioles
Polyarteritis nodosa (periarteritis)	Intima/media/ adventitia	Medium and small arteries
Syphilitic arteritis	Adventitia/media	Large and medium arteries
Giant-cell arteritis (allergic, granulomatous)	Media	Medium and small arteries

Epidemiological Considerations

Table II.
Average total number of deaths in the United States during one year (1974).*

Etiology	Number	Percent
Arterial diseases	874,000	45%
Cancer	336,000	18%
Accidents	155,000	6%
Respiratory diseases	113,000	5%
All other causes	490,000	26%

* Data obtained from the American Heart Association.

The interpretation of epidemiological data on the distribution of a multifactorial disease such as atherosclerosis is based on the evaluation of possible relationships between many environmental, genetic, and even social variables. It cannot, as has often been claimed, provide direct evidence of a cause-and-effect interaction for a single risk factor.

Epidemiological studies suffer the hazards of data collection by many investigators under varying conditions. An important contribution to standardized evaluation of arterial lesions and the geographic distribution of atherosclerosis was initiated in New Orleans in 1960 at the International Atherosclerosis Project (IAP). Examinations of aortas, coronary arteries, and, in some cases, cerebral vessels were carried out in over 20,000 samples collected in North, Central, and South America, and in Africa, Europe, and Southeast Asia. The extensive data obtained showed that the occurrence of raised arterial lesions ranged from a high of 18% for the white population in New Orleans to a low of 6% in African blacks. One important conclusion of the study was that populations with a higher incidence of raised aortic lesions also showed a higher incidence of extensive coronary atheroma.

The following are the most evident of all the consistent associations found:

Age: In all groups studied, severity and extent of both aortic and coronary atherosclerosis increase with age. However, there are significant variations in the severity of complicated lesions and resultant symptomatology. A more recent evaluation of data on male subjects, aged 10 to 39, from six locations in the IAP study, has shown that the extent of raised lesions in older patients is influenced by the histological characteristics (cellularity and foci of necrosis) of fatty streaks found in younger subjects from the same groups. Young black men had more extensive aortic fatty streaks than did other populations studied. However, this was not reflected in increased severity of raised lesions in older age groups.

In man, in contrast to other animals, the aging process induces specific changes of the arterial wall, particularly uniform intimal thickening. Aging influences atherogenesis mainly by increasing the effect of all other risk factors on the arterial wall (see the section on CURRENT CONCEPTS).

Sex: While coronary atherosclerosis appears more severe in men than in premenopausal women, the difference seems to be limited to the white populations studied. Several investigations have shown that black Americans and Africans do not show a marked sex difference in severity of coronary lesions.

The relationship between sex and atherogenesis seems to be far more complex than originally anticipated. This has been shown by the increased incidence of severe symptomatic coronary artery disease in premenopausal women who are heavy cigarette smokers as well as by the risk associated with lipid abnormalities induced by estrogens in birth-control medications. Extensive epidemiological studies carried out in Framingham, Massachusetts, have shown that in the United States, symptomatic coronary artery disease appears, on the average, ten years later in women than in men. If the comparison is based on proven myocardial infarctions, this difference between the sexes is increased to approximately 20 years.

Race: The significance of racial differences in atherogenesis reflects the genetic background of different populations and varies with the location of lesions. In general, coronary atherosclerosis is less severe in blacks than in whites. It develops in the black population, with the notable exception of black females in New Orleans, approximately a decade behind that of the white population.

These racial differences do not apply, however, to symptomatic peripheral atherosclerosis, particularly of cerebral vessels. The IAP study showed that blacks in New Orleans and Jamaica had consistently more atherosclerosis in intracranial and extracranial arteries than did whites; whites showed more aortic and coronary atherosclerosis. The findings correlate well with differences in mortality rates for cerebrovascular and coronary heart disease found between the races and the higher incidence of hypertension reported in blacks at all ages.

The IAP study clearly showed that, in both blacks and whites, atherosclerotic involvement was significantly higher in North America than in similar groups from Central and South America. These geographic differences in lesion distribution within similar ethnic groups strongly suggest that environmental conditions may exert considerably more influence than do racial characteristics on symptomatic atherosclerosis.

The increased severity and extent of arterial lesions in certain geographic areas are also reflected in mortality rates due to cardiovascular diseases. As indicated in Table II, arterial disease is the major cause of death in the United States. The figures do not accurately represent the incidence of coronary atherosclerosis in the general population, since many of these lesions remain subclinical or asymptomatic for long periods.

Structural and Functional Characteristics of the Normal Arterial Wall

Although cerebral vascular insufficiency and hypertension are considered to be at least five times more common in black men than in white, the latter have a 20% greater chance of dying of myocardial infarction than do their black counterparts. In black women, the risk of dying from coronary heart disease (CHD) is twice as high as for white women. This may be explained by the higher incidence of diabetes mellitus and hypercholesterolemia found in black women. The "racial" susceptibility to CHD seems, however, to result from environmental changes rather than the phenotypic expression of inherited racial characteristics. Support for this concept has been provided by large population studies carried out with Orientals living in San Francisco and Hawaii. Like other ethnic groups in the United States, they show a higher incidence of CHD than does the population in the country of their origin. As suggested by Dobzansky:

Equality is a social doctrine and variation is the biological norm. The overwhelming determinant of the variable human form and response is not genetic but environmental. Indeed, the variability of environment to which humans are exposed is the conspicuous and challenging social reality of our times.

Table III presents data from a study that compared the occurrence of atherosclerotic coronary artery disease (CAD) and ischemic heart disease (IHD) in a random sample of autopsy studies of 1,000 asymptomatic men between 45 and 65 years of age. In spite of extensive coronary pathology, only 20% of these cases showed morphological evidence of myocardial ischemia. Although the number of cases studied is too small to allow any definite conclusions, the data show that myocardial ischemia does not unavoidably follow severe coronary atherosclerosis and that epidemiological studies based on mortality statistics may be misleading regarding the overall incidence of CAD in a given population.

Table III.
Data indicating the relationship between the occurrence of coronary artery disease* and ischemic heart disease.†

Randomized autopsy findings in 1,000 asymptomatic men from 45 to 65 years of age

Almost 100% had coronary atherosclerosis

About 33% had over 50% anatomical stenosis of one or more coronary arteries

About 20% had ischemic myocardial pathology

About 15% had one occluded coronary artery

* **Coronary artery disease** (CAD) refers to a variety of pathological changes in the coronary arteries resulting in stenosis and eventual occlusion of the vascular lumen. Its most common etiology is coronary atherosclerosis.
† **Ischemic heart disease** (IHD) refers to any type of focal myocardial pathology induced by functional and/or anatomic reductions of blood and oxygen supply to the myocardium. CAD is by far its most common cause, but other disease processes may also play a role (see p. 47).

The arterial wall is a complex and highly structured organ. As illustrated in Figure 1, a medium-sized muscular or distributing vessel, such as a main coronary artery, consists of a series of coaxial tubes or tissue layers of specialized cells and extracellular components ideally suited for specific hemodynamic functions. In large arteries, there are three clearly defined layers: *tunica intima, tunica media,* and *tunica adventitia.*

The innermost layer of the intima, or endothelium, is in direct contact with circulating blood; it consists of specialized polygonal cells forming an essentially continuous cell monolayer that measures from 0.5 to 1.2 μ in thickness. *En face* staining techniques and electron microscopic studies have shown that these cells are arranged in characteristic mosaic configurations with occasional giant cells. The permeability characteristics of this cell layer to circulating macromolecules play a key role in the metabolism of the underlying arterial wall and seem to vary significantly between blood vessels. There are thought to be two major pathways by which substances enter the arterial wall through the normal endothelium. Larger molecules gain entry via pinocytotic or endocytotic vesicles, similar to the "large pore" system found in capillaries. By contrast, small particles, which vary in size and complexity, are believed to pass between cells at intercellular junctions. The latter route corresponds to the "small pore" system identified by physiologists some time ago. Although seemingly of little functional significance under normal conditions, interendothelial transport may play an important role in the initial stages of atherogenesis in the presence of vasoactive agents at sites of accelerated endothelial cell turnover (see the section on CURRENT CONCEPTS). Characteristically, the endothelial lining of normal arteries is quite smooth and regular, even at sites of branching (Figure 2), without attachment of circulating blood elements to its surface.

A distinct basement membrane, 200 to 300 mμ thick, separates the endothelium from the subendothelial space. At birth, the endothelial layer of human arteries rests directly against the fenestrated internal elastic membrane. It is only after the first decade of life that subendothelial elements become apparent. In contrast to other animals, the *tunica intima* of the adult human aorta reaches 1 mm or more in thickness. It contains polygonal cells with ultrastructural characteristics of vascular smooth muscle (intimacytes or myointimal cells) interlaced with bundles of collagen and elastin fibers and occasional fibroblasts.

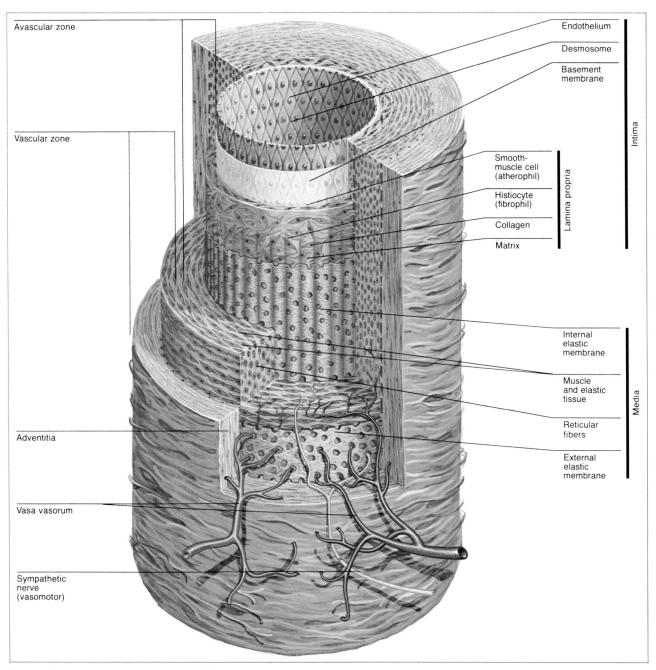

Avascular zone

Vascular zone

Adventitia

Vasa vasorum

Sympathetic
nerve
(vasomotor)

Endothelium

Desmosome

Basement
membrane

Intima

Smooth-
muscle cell
(atherophil)

Histiocyte
(fibrophil)

Collagen

Matrix

Lamina propria

Internal
elastic
membrane

Muscle
and elastic
tissue

Reticular
fibers

External
elastic
membrane

Media

Figure 1. Schematic structural characteristics of the
normal arterial wall.

Structural and Functional Characteristics of the Atherosclerotic Arterial Wall

Figure 2. Scanning electron micrograph of normal aortic endothelium at site of an intercostal branch (X 550). Please compare to Figure 10.

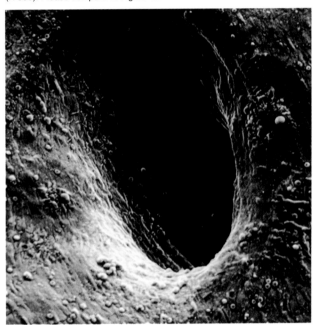

The *tunica media* is poorly demarcated from the intima in large arteries, since the internal elastic membrane is only the first of many similarly fenestrated elastic layers 6 to 19 μ apart, which are interconnected by elastic fibers. In the spaces between these layers, circumferentially arranged, elongated, smooth-muscle cells are present. Individual cells are surrounded by a network of thin collagenous and elastic fibers that bind them to the elastic membranes.

The *tunica adventitia* is relatively thin and is separated from the *media* by the external elastic membrane. This layer in large arteries contains small vessels called the *vasa vasora*, which are derived from branches of the main artery. These vessels form a complex capillary plexus in the external media. Small fascicles of unmyelinated nerve fibers, which contain abundant mitochondria and terminal synaptic vesicles, are also found in close proximity to the external elastic membrane (*vasa nervosa*).

The *tunica adventitia* merges gradually with the surrounding connective tissue without clearly defined boundaries, facilitating the changes in vascular diameter induced by the pulsatile blood flow.

INITIAL OR "EARLY" LESIONS

We have said before that perhaps the most striking characteristic of adult atherosclerosis is its pleomorphism, suggesting several episodic, and often synergistic, arterial reactions to injury.

Obviously, an indispensable requirement for developing specific therapeutic measures is to identify the initial stages of atherogenesis. Unfortunately, the term *early lesion* is often used to indicate either (1) minimally detectable variations from normal in the arterial wall, or (2) the arterial changes appearing in childhood that may theoretically evolve into the complicated lesions occurring in adults.

Confusion results because there is not an exclusive initial or early lesion. Such lesions are often found, interspersed with advanced atheroma, in adult patients. It seems reasonable, therefore, to describe them as initial lesions and classify and qualify them as follows:

1 Juvenile intimal thickening (mesenchymal cushions, fibromuscular intimal thickening)

This condition is found in the coronary arteries of all young humans, regardless of environmental or genetic influences. The thickened intimal layer consists of longitudinal arrays of modified smooth-muscle cells (intimacytes), increased ground substance, and collagen and elastic fibers, particularly at sites of arterial branching. These "cushions" appear in the abdominal aorta by the end of the first decade and considerably later in the thoracic segment. In infants and young children, cell proliferation is a prominent characteristic of lesions. In adolescents, focal intracellular lipid deposits are common.

Although these coronary artery lesions are often more extensive in male than in female infants, their role as precursors of adult coronary atheroma has yet to be demonstrated. Most investigators believe that they are examples of localized areas of vascular remodeling resulting from changes in blood flow during development (Figure 3).

2 Fatty streaks

This term has been used to describe all flat or slightly raised intimal lesions containing abundant intracellular or extracellular lipids; epidemiological and experimental studies suggest that several subtypes may be present:

a) Juvenile fatty streaks: Characteristically, these are found in childhood and adolescence as grossly visible round or oval lesions containing sudanophilic lipids. Microscopi-

Figure 3. Early lesions in human arteries (oil red "O" surface stain).

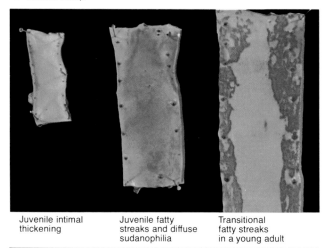

Juvenile intimal thickening | Juvenile fatty streaks and diffuse sudanophilia | Transitional fatty streaks in a young adult

cally, lipid-laden modified smooth-muscle cells, or intimacytes, are surrounded by connective tissue elements in the absence of extracellular lipid pools. Unlike other atherosclerotic lesions, they are more common in black than in white populations and are more extensive in women.

b) *Transitional fatty streaks:* These appear in young adults and are predominant in populations that have a high frequency of symptomatic atherosclerosis. They are found in the coronary arteries by the end of the second decade. Unlike fatty streaks in the abdominal aorta, which usually appear earlier, these coronary lesions increase in severity as the patient ages and by the third and fourth decades are found mixed with fibrous plaques. By then, they also appear in peripheral arteries, including those of the cerebral circulation. Histologically, transitional fatty streaks contain abundant extracellular lipids resulting from degeneration and necrosis of lipid-laden cells.

This type of fatty streak is considered to be the initial lesion of atherosclerosis and is believed to have the potential to evolve into the atherosclerotic plaques found in adult patients.

c) *Regressive fatty streaks:* These fatty lesions are found in elderly persons. They are characterized by diffuse infiltration of membrane-bound extracellular lipid vacuoles, in the immediate vicinity of the internal elastic membrane surrounded by altered elastic and collagen fibers. Since similar lesions have been found in experimental models after discontinuing atherogenic regimens, these fatty streaks in man are thought to be examples of various stages of regression from more severe lesions.

One important biochemical characteristic of all human fatty streaks is the predominance of cholesterol and its esters as the major lipid components of the lesions. It is believed that most of the cholesterol within arterial lesions is derived from the plasma lipoproteins. In contrast to more advanced atherosclerotic lesions, the cholesteryl ester of fatty streaks contains a high proportion of cholesteryl oleate. An interpretation of this finding is that, although the sterol moiety comes from the blood, the fatty acid components of the ester are synthesized locally by cells found in the transitional fatty streaks. An imbalance between the rate of cholesteryl esterification and hydrolysis presumably occurs within the arterial wall. (See section CURRENT CONCEPTS: The Role of the Arterial Cell.)

Most fatty streaks also contain variable amounts of connective tissue components, including collagen, elastin, glycosaminoglycans, and glycoproteins. These substances may play an important role in altering the transport and "trapping" circulating macromolecules, particularly lipoproteins, across the arterial wall. Quantitative and structural variations in these vascular components during the initial stages of atherogenesis are under intensive investigation, since they undoubtedly play a key role in the evolution of fatty streaks into adult-type lesions.

3 Gelatinous or insudation lesions

Although these lesions may morphologically resemble a juvenile fatty streak, they are characterized by large concentrations of extracellular glycosaminoglycans and perifibrous lipid droplets associated with fragmented elastic fibers. They have been found only in the aorta. Their lipid pattern resembles that of low-density lipoproteins (LDL), with linoleate rather than oleate as the major component of its cholesteryl esters. Whether or not these lesions have a different origin than fatty streaks and how they relate to the adult-type atheroma has yet to be established.

FIBROUS PLAQUES

There is considerable disagreement regarding the relationship, if any, of these lesions with those previously described. It is believed that they are often preceded by transitional fatty streaks.

The term *fibrous plaque* is used to describe a variety of morphological and biochemical changes of the arterial wall.

44

Figure 4A. Complicated artherosclerotic lesion of a main right coronary artery showing characteristic intimal changes resulting in severe stenosis.

Figure 4B. Complete occlusion of main coronary artery, showing extensive lipid infiltrates and marginal recanalization. (Frozen section, Sudan IV stain; X 100.)

A

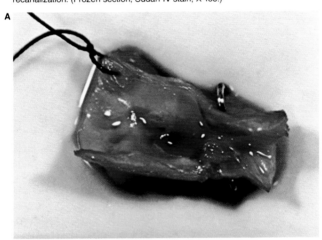

B

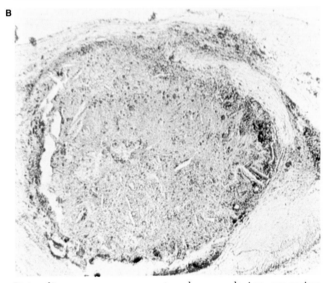

core of variable size, surrounded by a thick capsule of collagenous and elastic tissue containing abundant glycosaminoglycans and glycoproteins. The composition of this lipid core closely resembles that of blood plasma, with a high concentration of linoleate rather than oleate in its cholesteryl esters. It has been suggested that this implies increased permeability of fibrous plaques to plasma components, in agreement with the higher uptake of labeled albumin or lipoprotein fractions observed in experimental lesions.

COMPLICATED LESIONS

These are the most common types of atherosclerotic lesions that produce significant circulatory changes and clinical symptoms in the adult population. They may induce severe (Figure 4a) or even complete obstruction (Figure 4b) of the arterial lumen, with subsequent ischemia or infarction.

Complicated lesions usually develop from preexisting fibro-fatty lesions, as a result of one or a combination of several histological changes:

1 Necrosis and pultaceous softening that is often followed by disruption of the lesion with release of fatty materials and cell debris into the circulation, leaving an ulceration.

2 Mural thrombi, occurring particularly at sites of ulceration, may evolve into complete thrombosis with secondary canalization. Acute occlusive thrombosis at the site of a preexisting lesion is the most common source of clinical manifestations.

3 Intramural hematomas, often accompanied by discrete areas of inflammatory cell infiltrates, with increased *vasa vasora* and ground matrix that may eventually evolve into mural thrombi.

4 Hemorrhage and occasional dissection of the ulcerated plaque, usually around areas of calcification.

One important hemodynamic characteristic of complicated lesions, particularly those with amorphous deposits of dystrophic calcification in an avascular fibrous matrix, is loss of elasticity as compared with the normal arterial wall. When accompanied by thinning and atrophy of the muscular medial layer, these changes facilitate development of aneurysmal dilatations and even eventual rupture.

DEVELOPMENT OF LESIONS AT CELL LEVEL

As previously indicated, the development of spontaneous atherosclerosis into the adult lesion is a very slow process, usually requiring several decades to exhibit clinical symptoms. The cellular changes found in an artery are therefore

It implies a more permanent and severe lesion appearing later in life. In contrast to fatty streaks, fibrous plaques closely follow the development of clinical atherosclerosis in distribution and severity.

In susceptible populations, fibrous plaques first appear at sites of branching in the abdominal aorta in young adults and in the coronary arteries by the end of the third decade. Shortly thereafter, they are found in other peripheral arteries, including those of the cerebral circulation.

Fibrous plaques are characterized histologically by a lipid

Figure 5. Four histological regions in the development of an atherosclerotic human lesion.

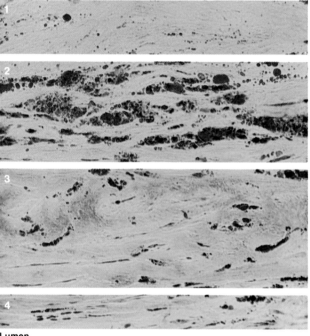

Lumen

1. Injury (early changes)
2. Proliferation (intracellular lipids)
3. Necrosis (extracellular lipids)
4. Repair (fibrous cap)

Table IV.
Pathological sequence of human atherosclerosis.

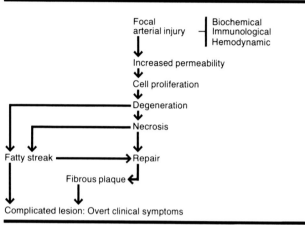

related to the biological age of individual lesions, rather than the stage of the overall disease process.

Figure 5 is a histological section of a typical atherosclerotic lesion in the carotid artery of a 42-year-old patient with diffuse vascular disease. Arbitrary lines have been drawn to indicate approximately four different histological regions, which exemplify the four stages of arterial cell involvement that have been identified both clinically and experimentally as characteristic of atherogenesis.

Stage 1: Injury
A variety of insults constantly challenge the arterial wall, resulting in focal increases in permeability to circulating macromolecules, thickening of the subendothelial space, and secondary cell proliferation (see Table IV).

Stage 2: Proliferation
Proliferation of intimacytes or intimal smooth-muscle cells is accompanied by significant alteration of arterial cell metab-

olism, resulting in the appearance of intracellular lipid vacuoles rich in cholesteryl esters. The intimacytes then become "foam" cells, or atherocytes. These begin to show both histochemical and ultrastructural degenerative changes, leading to stage 3.

Stage 3: Necrosis
Irreversible cell damage, with lysis and release of intracellular contents, causes large accumulations of extracellular lipids and connective-tissue changes characteristic of the initiation of stage 4.

Stage 4: Repair
Repair, with deposition of collagen and elastin fibers and scattered fibroblastic elements, leads to the characteristic connective tissue changes described in the section on Fibrous Plaques and to secondary development of the complicated lesion.

It should be reemphasized that, in any susceptible adult artery, it is often possible to identify lesions at one or more of the histological stages described (Figure 6). *This is conceptually important for the initiation of therapeutic measures to prevent progression of the disease.*

THE ARTERIAL SMOOTH-MUSCLE CELL
In large- and medium-sized arteries, medial smooth-muscle cells are the most common cellular components of the arterial wall. Since Haust and More, as well as Geer et al, described cells with morphological and histochemical characteristics

Figure 6. Proliferative stage of atherosclerosis; shown are predominant intimal thickening and alterations of the internal elastic membrane. (Masson's trichrome stain; X 240.)

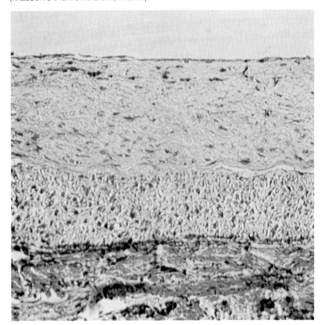

of smooth muscle in "early" lesions, a great number of studies in experimental models of atherosclerosis have confirmed and extended their observations.

Wissler and co-workers have emphasized the multifunctional potentials of medial smooth-muscle cells as the mesenchymal components able to synthesize collagen, elastin, and ground substance in the vessel wall. They also showed that these cells are able to proliferate and migrate under a variety of stimuli, including specific lipoprotein fractions, as is the case with similar cells found in the thickened human arterial intima (see the section on CURRENT CONCEPTS).

Ross and associates have provided further evidence of the wide capabilities of vascular smooth muscle with their studies on the effects of platelet factors on growth rates and synthesis of connective tissue elements by monkey medial cells *in vitro.*

In human lesions, there is no doubt that cells fulfilling ultrastructural criteria of smooth muscle are present in areas of intimal thickening. They share many functional similarities with the overlying endothelial cells, and their origin is still under investigation. It has recently been suggested that endothelial and smooth-muscle cells in large arteries may share a common ancestry, representing specialized transitional stages of metabolically and functionally similar cell populations.

The morphological identification of such cells as *endothelial, smooth muscle, fibroblast,* or *macrophage* provides traditional histological labels of limited functional significance. In order to avoid preconceived notions about their origin, we have proposed the term *intimacyte* to describe any cell found in the adult human intima with the characteristics of vascular smooth muscle. We have further identified such cells in transitional fatty streaks as *atherophils* or *atherocytes,* depending on their intracellular lipid content (see the section on CURRENT CONCEPTS).

DISTRIBUTION OF ATHEROMATA
IN RELATION TO SEVERITY OF SYMPTOMS

In large blood vessels, atherosclerotic lesions predominantly occur at sites of bifurcation and at the origin of branch vessels. Within different arteries, and even within different segments of the same artery, there may be considerable variation in the severity of lesions. This selective localization is frequently apparent in the iliac arteries. Stenosis is most common in the internal iliac arteries and least common in the external iliacs; the common iliacs occupy an intermediate position. The left common iliac artery is unique in that stenoses are most frequent in its proximal third. In contrast, the right and left internal iliacs, the external iliacs, and the right common iliac arteries show no preference for such segmental lesion distribution. This interesting difference between the right and left common iliac arteries is probably due to hemodynamic changes resulting from variation in the angle of origin of these two vessels from the aorta.

In arteries of the lower extremities, narrowing or occlusion may be quite localized, or, more commonly, multisegmental. Physical or mechanical injury may aid not only in determining plaque localization but also in initiating thrombosis. Two such vulnerable sites are the *adductus magnus* opening, where the femoral artery may be subject to compression and angulation, and just above the knee joint, where the popliteal artery is prone to severe repetitive injuries. Atherosclerosis and thrombosis are also commonly found in the femoral artery within the femoral canal, another site where recurrent mechanical injury may be a factor.

Angiographic techniques for arterial visualization have shown that, in the lower extremities, occlusions most frequently occur in the tibial-peroneal arteries (26.5%) and in

Figure 7. Relationship of severity of coronary artery disease to degree of arterial obstruction.

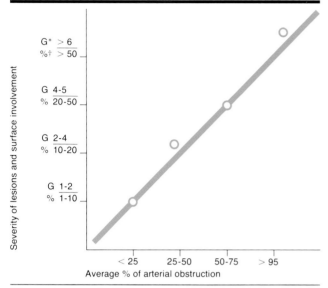

*G = grade or severity of lesion
†% = surface involvement

the femoral-popliteal-tibial system either with (26.9%) or without (22.2%) associated aortoiliac disease.

The distribution of atherosclerotic lesions in the coronary arteries is rather characteristic. In the anterior descending branch of the left coronary artery, lesions are usually present in the first 2 to 3 cm distal to its aortic orifice and in the circumflex branch at a point just beyond its origin from the main trunk. In the right coronary artery, major lesions are usually found within the first 3 to 5 cm from its point of origin in the ascending aorta.

Extensive atherosclerosis of multiple coronary branches is frequently found in older patients, whereas symptomatic coronary artery disease (CAD) in patients of both sexes under age 50 is often the result of a severe single stenotic coronary lesion correctable by surgery. Single stenotic lesions often cause anterior myocardial infarction, but in patients with acute posterior infarcts, stenotic lesions are often present in all three main coronary arteries. The functional significance of severe stenotic lesions varies between coronary branches; such lesions often induce symptoms earlier when present in the left anterior descending than in the circumflex or in the right coronary arteries. Unfortunately, x-ray visualization of severe calcification in these lesions does not accurately measure stenotic involvement of the vessels. Coronary cineangiography must be used to evaluate the degree of arterial obstruction.

The relationship between severity of coronary artery disease and arterial stenosis is shown graphically in Figure 7. It clearly demonstrates that, as coronary artery lesions increase in size and depth, there is an exponential elevation in severity of arterial obstruction. Vessels with lesions above grade 6 and with over 50% surface involvement are completely occluded.

MYOCARDIAL ISCHEMIA AND MYOCARDIAL INFARCTION

The usual consequence of stenotic coronary atherosclerosis is an inadequacy of blood and oxygen supply to the myocardium, inducing symptoms of myocardial ischemia or ischemic heart disease (IHD).*

If severe ischemia is the result of acute and total coronary occlusion, myocardial infarction will ensue. This will not necessarily be the final outcome if the occlusion develops gradually. Collateral circulation may take over, allowing nourishment of the heart muscle, in spite of multiple occluded coronary vessels. It is a common clinical belief that the severity of angina pectoris is proportional to the degree of coronary artery disease and relative ischemia of the distal myocardium. If acute coronary thrombosis has occurred, and the patient has survived the stress of acute myocardial ischemia, organization of the thrombus ensues, followed usually by canalization. The compromised coronary vessel is able to carry only a limited amount of blood to the distal heart muscle, maintaining a restricted myocardial function.*

The area of ischemic necrosis may vary in size from focal (and often microscopic) to diffuse and massive. Most grossly visible infarcts measure from 1 to 5 cm in width and do not involve the myocardial wall uniformly. The infarcts may be subendocardial and accompanied by mural thrombi in one area, while transmural in another area. When the subepicardial muscle is involved, fibrinous pericarditis may follow.

The most frequent site for myocardial infarcts is the anterior aspect of the interventricular septum, extending to the anterior third of the lateral wall and apical portions of the left ventricle, as the result of acute occlusion of the descending branch of the left coronary artery. The second-most common area is the posterior third of the septum and the basal or posterior aspect of the left ventricle; here the infarct is due to occlusion of the right coronary. If infarction is first confined to the lateral wall of the left ventricle, it is usually due to occlusion of the left circumflex artery. Acute obstruction of the left or right main coronary arteries is lethal if it occurs close to the aortic ostia. Isolated atrial infarcts occur rarely; they are associated with infarction of the ventricles. Although it has not been proven, it is believed that oxygenated blood from the left auricle tends to protect this cardiac chamber from infarction.

*Although coronary atherosclerosis is by far the most common cause of IHD, other diseases of the coronary arteries, such as granulomatous arteritis (Takayasu's), panarteritis of varied etiology, ankylosing spondylitis, and Hurler's syndrome, should also be considered. Furthermore, myocardial ischemia may occur in the absence of overt coronary artery pathology such as that found in Prinzmetal angina, thyrotoxicosis, cardiac myxomas, or congenital anomalies.

The gross appearance of a recent infarct is a purplish area with brownish mottling of the epicardium, which is often covered by a thin film of fibrin. Necrotic muscle fibers give the heart a light brown or yellow color on section. Patches of hemorrhagic discoloration are usually present at the edges.

Histological evidence of recent myocardial infarction may be difficult to find by routine methods if the patient died within five or six hours after acute occlusion. Table V summarizes the most characteristic histological and ultrastructural changes of a typical myocardial infarct relative to its biological age.

Differentiation from an old, healed, or fibrotic infarct is clear and unequivocal. If the myocardium is to continue functioning, scar tissue must replace the dead muscle. The time necessary for an infarct to heal depends on its size and on the amount of collateral circulation present. Small infarcts may heal in less than five weeks, and more extensive infarcts may take as long as two months. As shown in Table VI, common complications of myocardial infarction are often serious, ranging from rupture of the heart to endocardial damage, aneurysmal dilatation, or secondary pericarditis. When nonelastic fibrous tissue replaces the normal heart muscle, the wall of the heart, particularly of the left ventricle, tends to bulge or stretch under systolic pressure. This results in round, sac-like bulges in the cardiac silhouette. Surgical repair of these lesions has significantly reduced the mortality rate associated with such complications.

The most lethal result of myocardial infarction is heart rupture. It may occur in the anterior surface of the heart, as a result of an untreated ventricular aneurysm, or through the intraventricular septum, with serious hemodynamic consequences. Patients with severe systolic hypertension are three times more likely to develop cardiac rupture than are normotensive individuals.

As indicated above, infarction of the subendocardial muscle may induce formation of mural thrombi. Following secondary healing of the heart muscle, these may break free, causing distal embolization to peripheral organs, particularly the brain and the kidney. A similar mechanism may also cause rupture of a papillary muscle and the development of acute mitral insufficiency.

One fairly common complication of acute myocardial infarction is *pericarditis epistenocardiaca*. When a patient who has had an acute myocardial infarct suddenly develops recurrence of chest pains within ten days to two to three weeks after his heart attack, a postmyocardial infarction syndrome may be present. Differential diagnosis is aided by radiological demonstration of pulmonary infiltration and electrocardiographic changes compatible with pericarditis rather than with typical myocardial infarction.

Table V.
The histopathological stages of myocardial infarction.

1. 0 to 60 minutes	Subcellular changes of ischemic heart muscle (mitochondrial granules, reduction of glycogen and respiratory enzymes)
2. 1 to 6 hours	Margination and clumping of nuclear chromatin; loss of nuclear and myofilament architecture; infiltration with neutrophils
3. 6 to 12 hours	Typical ischemic necrosis: muscle pale, dry, and opaque, with poor demarcation; epicardium hemorrhagic and mottled
4. After 24 hours	Severe histological changes easily recognizable
5. 2 to 4 days	Focal hemorrhages of variable size; muscle pale; beginning of demarcation by jagged line of leukocytes surrounded by red band of dilated capillaries and hemorrhage
6. 6 to 8 days	Yellow, friable infarcted area due to fatty degeneration leads to aneurysm or rupture
7. 8 to 10 days	Depressed lesion due to removal of damaged muscle by phagocytosis; vascularized peripheral granulation tissue
8. 3 to 4 weeks	Granulation and fibrosis lead to scar formation
9. 2 to 3 months or longer	Healing process mostly completed, depending on size of infarct; eventual dystrophic calcification may occur

Table VI.
Effects of myocardial infarction.

1. Myocardial fibrosis	
2. Rupture of:	Heart Papillary muscle Interventricular septum
3. Endocardial damage:	Mural thrombus ↓ Distal embolism
4. Aneurysm of the heart	
5. Pericarditis epistenocardiaca (postmyocardial infarction syndrome)	

Current Concepts

THE ROLE OF ARTERIAL CELLS
IN THE DEVELOPMENT OF ATHEROSCLEROSIS

It should be emphasized that the complicated lesion found in adult human arteries is not the result of a single factor but of a constellation of etiological factors. Atherosclerosis may thus be defined as *an abnormal response of some areas of the vascular wall to the cumulative and often synergistic effects of episodic injury-repair processes, causing permanent arterial damage.*

In order to evaluate functional characteristics and metabolic requirements of human arterial cells, as well as their response to atherogenic risk factors, we have studied their behavior in cell and organ cultures since 1954. These investigations have shown that from the adult human arterial intima it is possible to isolate the intimacytes in culture as a well-defined cell population. These cells share some of the cytochemical, immunofluorescent, and ultrastructural characteristics of medial smooth-muscle cells described on pages 45 and 46. The other cellular components of the intima, the endothelia, while less numerous than the intimacytes in large arteries, have some subcellular components of both cell types. These findings are interpreted to indicate a common ancestry for all three cell types in the adult blood vessel. Figure 8 demonstrates the growth characteristics of coronary intimacytes after isolation by cloning. Unlike endothelial cells, intimacytes, after reaching confluence, tend to form cell aggregates or mounds with typical accumulation of glycosaminoglycans, elastin, and collagen.

One important phenotypic characteristic of intimacytes obtained from histologically disease-free areas of atherosclerotic arteries is shown in Figure 9. Intracellular uptake of labeled cholesterol from pooled homologous low-density lipoproteins was considerably higher than that of similar cells obtained from matching samples of atheroma-free arteries from patients of the same sex and age groups.

Other metabolic abnormalities of such cells are shown in Table VII. Diploid monoclonal cultures of coronary intimacytes incubated in 20% pooled type II hyperlipemic sera showed not only accelerated uptake of lipoprotein lipids but also a significant increase in intracellular cholesteryl esters compared with matching cell preparations incubated in normal sera. In contrast to skeletal muscle cells or adipocytes also tested, increased cell cholesteryl ester accumulation did not inhibit *de novo* synthesis of cholesterol from ^{14}C acetate in such cells. Absence of this key feedback mechanism regu-

Figure 8. Mass cell-culture technique of human intimacytes for analytical studies. Note abundant cell clones. (Unstained preparation, X 2.)

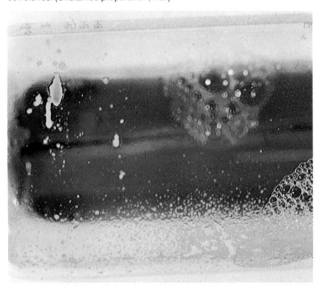

lating cholesterol synthesis in atherosclerotic artery intimacytes could explain the accelerated development of cholesteryl-ester-rich fatty lesions in early atherogenesis.

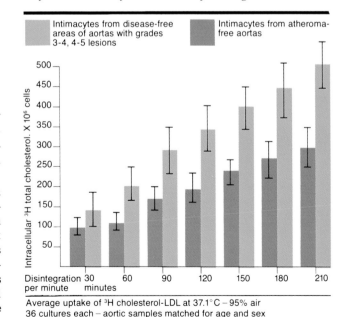

Average uptake of ^{3}H cholesterol-LDL at 37.1°C – 95% air
36 cultures each – aortic samples matched for age and sex

Figure 9. Differences in rates of cholesterol uptake of human aortic intimal cells *in vitro.*

These findings resemble the recent observations by Goldstein and Brown of LDL-deficient receptors in skin fibroblasts of patients with homozygous type II hyperlipoproteinemias and in the regulation of controlling enzymes for cholesterol biosynthesis by mesenchymal cells.

Another important area of current research is growth stimulation of arterial cells by lipoprotein fractions and platelet-rich plasma in cell culture. Experimental findings to date suggest that low-density lipoprotein fractions from type II hyperlipemic sera and platelet factors enhance arterial cell proliferation.

Benditt and associates have recently investigated the origin of cells found in human fibrous plaques. The enzyme pattern found within the lesions suggested that the cells had orginated from a single cell type. The term *monoclonal* was used to describe the single origin of such cells, which result from arterial cell proliferation. Such a monoclonal population could develop by cell transformation as a result of chemical or viral mutagens, with selectional advantage for a specific cell type. The growth of an atheromatous plaque could thus be considered similar to the development of a benign vascular tumor. This challenging concept is summarized in Table VIII relative to the stages of human atherogenesis.

Another cellular element of the arterial wall, which is receiving increased attention, is the endothelium. Investigators are examining its important regulatory function on arterial wall permeability. Although normal endothelial cells of large arteries provide a continually impervious layer to circulating macromolecules and blood cells, a variety of vasoactive stimuli from hormones to platelets may temporarily alter this layer's permeability. We have proposed the term *trap door effect* to describe it. The pathophysiological significance of these findings on the initial stages of atherogenesis is under close scrutiny.

By and large, all types of spontaneous atherosclerosis in wild animals are significantly less severe. Animals develop symptomatic lesions much less frequently than does man. This may be partly related to the unusual anatomical and functional characteristics of the vascular wall of large- and medium-sized human arteries. These arteries are supplied with nutrients from two sources: (1) the intima and inner media by direct perfusion of metabolites from the vascular lumen, and (2) the outer media and adventitia by a complex net of small arterioles and venules, the *vasa vasora* (see Figure 1). The watershed, or avascular zone, between these two

Table VII.
Human coronary artery intimal cells; diploid monoclonal intimacytes. Changes in intracellular lipid concentrations and *de novo* sterol synthesis following incubation in media containing 20% pooled normolipemic (1) or hyperlipemic human sera (2).

Total lipids	NS(1)	HS(2)
Triglycerides	44*	108
Free cholesterol	86	194
Cholesteryl esters	28	482
FC/CE ratios	3.07	0.40
Synthetized FC/CE†		
Average percent total sterols	79/21	18/82
Average dpm/μg sterols	640/64	28/287
1. Normolipemic sera = (mg/100 ml)	TC:208 CE:104	TG:84 PH:264
2. Type II hyperlipoproteinemias = (mg/100 ml)	TC:396 CE:294	TG:104 PH:290

* Average results in μg lipids/mg cell protein after 60-minute incubation at 37°C.
† From ^{14}C acetate.

Table VIII.
Hypothesis on cytogenetic changes in the etiology of human atherosclerosis.*

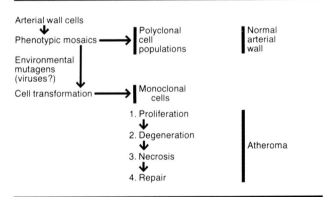

*Modified from Benditt EP, Benditt JM: *Proc Natl Acad Sci U.S.A.* 70:1753, 1973.

metabolic supplies is easily affected by changes in perfusion pressure resulting from hemodynamic alterations in the vascular lumen. Such changes may occur following increase in thickness and/or reduction of permeability of the arterial intima. Deposition of blood components such as platelets and/or fibrin on the endothelial surface may follow mechanical injury of the vascular wall due to turbulence, wave reflection, or shearing effects of the pulse wave, particularly at sites of arterial branching. These factors may also induce the development of focal areas of hypoxia and may significantly alter the metabolism and transport of macromolecules across the arterial wall, causing trapping of lipoproteins in the avascular region. Metabolic and rheological changes of the arterial wall may initiate this process of injury and repair; some immunological responses, such as allograft rejection, also seem to dramatically accelerate spontaneous atheroma.

PATHOGENESIS

There are almost as many hypotheses on the pathogenesis of atherosclerosis in man as there are investigators studying it. One important theory that has been proposed is referred to as the *filtration theory*. Based on considerable experimental data, the hypothesis is that plasma components, particularly lipids dissociated from blood lipoproteins, are trapped following filtration from the lumen in the inner intima and media (the metabolic watershed referred to earlier). Following lipid uptake by intimacytes, ground substance changes appear, particularly alterations in glycosaminoglycans. The latter bind lipid and lipoproteins and induce the increased metachromasia often observed in early fatty lesions.

As an alternative, some investigators have recently revived the concept of intramural hemorrhage first proposed by Paterson (1936) in the genesis of coronary occlusion. It is not yet clear whether or not hemorrhage precedes plaque formation and, as suggested by Winternitz (1938), is a source of lipid for raised arterial lesions, or results from tears on the stiff surface of a plaque. Other factors also influence the development of complicated coronary lesions: medial thinning, gross loss and disorganization of elastic tissue, and adventitial inflammatory changes.

A more likely possibility is the role of mural and transient deposition of platelet aggregates, following changes in platelet stickiness on the endothelial surface. The role of fibrinolysin and other proteolytic enzymes in maintaining homeostasis of normal endothelium, and their possible failure in atherosclerosis, may also be important secondary etiological factors.

The well-developed atherosclerotic plaque, resulting from the interplay of inflammatory and reparative processes, is a complex lesion containing extracellular deposits of calcium salts, blood components, cholesterol crystals, and glycosaminoglycans. The latter may be of great significance in regulat-

ing the transport of macromolecules from the extracellular compartment to the cytoplasm of vascular cells. It has been shown that anionic substances, such as some glycosaminoglycans in the ground substance, significantly inhibit transport of macromolecules across the cell membrane. This regulatory function of ground substance components may be important not only in atherogenesis but also in vascular inflammation. The initial changes, however, seem to occur at the cell level. Electron microscopy has shown that such changes are often accompanied by abnormal intracellular storage of lipids, particularly cholesteryl esters, fatty acids, and lipoprotein complexes. These findings have strengthened the thesis that lipid infiltration from the bloodstream may be a significant factor in the growth of, but not necessarily in the cause of, the initial atheromatous plaque.

INFLUENCE OF OTHER FACTORS
ON THE PATHOGENESIS OF ATHEROSCLEROSIS

The role of environmental risk factors is discussed in detail in SECTION I, thus the following review will be limited to factors contributing to the pathogenesis of atherosclerosis.

Patients with sustained hypertension are at greater risk of developing severe atherosclerosis than are normotensives. It is interesting that diastolic blood pressure levels have been correlated with fibrous plaque severity in men but not in women. The reason for this sex difference is unknown. Diastolic blood pressure, on the other hand, does not correlate with severity of complicated lesions in either gender, reflecting the heterogenous character of these lesions regardless of sex influences.

It is not clear if renovascular and essential hypertension play similar roles in the development of accelerated atherosclerosis, nor do we know how significant their atherogenic effects are in the absence of serum lipid abnormalities. However, there is no doubt that, in the general population, hypertensives have a higher incidence of ischemic heart attacks and cerebral vascular insufficiency. It is also well established that, although intimal changes are universally found in the pulmonary arteries of patients over age 40, pulmonary hypertension is a prerequisite for the development of severe and often complicated atheroma in the main pulmonary vessels.

Increased rates of development of complicated atherosclerotic lesions due to hemorrhage, ulceration, or thrombosis are common in hypertensives. Such patients also show a greater tendency for rupture of intracranial arteries. The latter may

Table IX.
Incorporation of tritiated lipoprotein fractions by rat aortic intima*
after endothelial stimulation with angiotensin II.†

Percent of radioactivity from plasma		Simultaneous injection with angiotensin II	Injected 60 sec after angiotensin II	Injected 480 sec after angiotensin II
VLDL		7.8	5.4	—
	S‡	1.24	1.82	—
LDL		16.2	8.4	0.4
	S̄	4.64	1.49	—
HDL		4.3	0.4	—
	S̄	1.47	0.12	—

* Intima and inner medial layers.
† Left intraventricular injection of 0.1 ng angiotensin II in 0.2 ml Ringer's solution in a 200-gm Sprague-Dawley rat.
‡ S̄ = Standard deviation of the mean.

Table X.
Current cardiovascular incidence in the United States.

Prevalence

Over 27 million with cardiovascular disease (CVD)
Over 22 million with high blood pressure (HBP)
Over 3.5 million with ischemic heart disease (IHD)
Over 1.5 million with rheumatic heart disease (RHD)
Over 1.5 million with cerebral vascular insufficiency (CVI)

Some major risk factors

High blood pressure*	increases risk of myocardial infarction by 2:1 increases risk of cerebral vascular insufficiency by 4:1
Hyperlipidemia†	increases risk of myocardial infarction by 3:1
Smoking	increases risk of myocardial infarction by 2:1 increases risk of cerebral vascular insufficiency by 5:1

* See Section I, pp 27, 28.
† See Section I, Table IV.

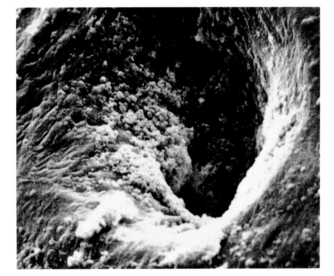

Figure 10. Scanning electron micrograph of aortic endothelium 40 seconds after intracardiac stimulation with epinephrine (X 550). Note "stickiness" of chylomicrons and platelets to the distal lip of the orifice of intercostal branch. Please compare with control, Figure 2.

often be the result of increased arterial fragility rather than perforation of a preexisting plaque. Good clinical and experimental data show that hemodynamic stresses are significantly increased by sustained systemic hypertension. Hypertension increases lateral pressure, turbulence, and limits arterial wall pliability, resulting in increased stiffness of the inner vascular layers. These rheological alterations exert a profound influence on the metabolism of the vessel wall and on its relationship to circulating macromolecules and blood cells.

In renovascular hypertension resulting from increased renin plasma levels, atherogenesis may be accelerated by increased arterial endothelial permeability as a result of the local effects of angiotensin II. Table IX shows increased trapping of lipoprotein fractions in the rat aortic intima after simultaneous stimulation with doses of angiotensin II insufficient to induce sustained, systemic hypertension. Because of the short half-life (30 to 45 seconds) of this vasoactive agent in the systemic circulation, delayed injections showed considerably fewer effects. Note that LDL uptake was significantly higher than either VLDL or HDL fractions. Figure 10 illustrates the effects of epinephrine (200 ng) injected in a normotensive rat, which caused chylomicrons and platelets to stick to the arterial surface at sites of rapid endothelial cell turnover.

Hypertension is a well-established risk factor for accelerated atherosclerosis in the adult. A prognostic relationship exists between severity of hypertension and life expectancy. This association is significantly aggravated in the young hypertensive if hyperlipidemia is also present.

It is significant that adequate therapy for hypertension in middle-aged patients reduces cerebral vascular accidents but does not influence coronary atherosclerosis. This suggests that detection and treatment of hypertension in the young is a pressing clinical objective for prevention of arterial disease.

The overall impact of cardiovascular disease in the United States is shown in Table X. It shows that hypertension is twice as severe a risk factor for CVI* as it is for myocardial infarction (MI) and that hyperlipemic patients have an incidence of MI three times higher than normolipemic individuals. Finally, cigarette smoking increases both CVI and MI in the overall population.

*The term CVI (cerebral vascular insufficiency) is preferred to the more commonly used CVA (cerebral vascular accident) since the latter is never an accident but a diagnosable and often preventable ischemic episode. (See Adelson L: Let's do away with CVA [letter to the editor]. JAMA 236:2390, 1976.)

Genetic and Environmental Factors

It is a deeply rooted tradition in medical education that by identifying the cause we can cure the illness. This principle has been highly successful in eradicating major infectious diseases in the past half-century. It may, however, have limited application in curing complex multifactorial disorders such as atherosclerosis, where environmental, metabolic, and genetic factors interact in the development of overt disease.

In the previous sections, we have attempted to show that symptomatic atherosclerosis, an endemic and lethal disease of modern man, is plurifactorial in origin and multiform in character. It affects all large arteries, but its clinical significance depends on location and severity of circulatory changes induced by luminal narrowing.

A summary of the influence of known risk factors for coronary artery disease is presented in Table XI. It shows that genetic risk factors, such as arterial wall susceptibility to atherogenesis, diabetes, and hyperlipoproteinemias, acting alone or in combination with those metabolic changes induced or expressed in adult life, may accelerate coronary atherogenesis.

The influence of environmental and genetic factors in atheroma development is summarized in Figure 11. The role of genetic traits in hereditary disorders such as phenylketonuria and galactosemia is shown at one end of the curve; the effects of environmental factors in industrial diseases are shown at the other end. Metabolic diseases such as atherosclerosis and diabetes are in the middle of the diagram. Although phenotypic expression of a polygenic trait for such common disorders seems epidemiologically present, environmental risk factors often exist in symptomatic patients.

These risk factors, while unable to significantly alter susceptibility to atherosclerosis in a given population, may indeed be significant in accelerating the development of symptomatic complicated lesions.

Definitive evidence that reducing risk factors will prevent development of spontaneous atheroma in man is lacking; however, considerable epidemiological and experimental evidence suggests that their prevention may retard the progression of lesions to the complicated (symptomatic) stage. It follows, therefore, that preventive measures should be taken prior to the critical time when adult lesions develop.

Table XI.
Some risk factors influencing the pathogenesis of atherosclerosis.

Congenital	Arterial cell susceptibility
	Diabetes
	Familial hyperlipoproteinemias
Acquired	Hypertension
	Smoking
	Secondary hyperlipoproteinemia
	Stress – hemodynamic changes

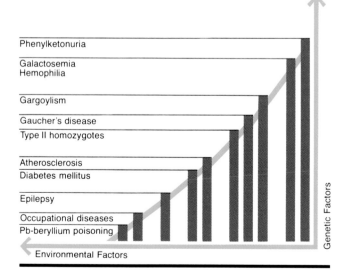

Phenylketonuria
Galactosemia
Hemophilia
Gargoylism
Gaucher's disease
Type II homozygotes
Atherosclerosis
Diabetes mellitus
Epilepsy
Occupational diseases
Pb-beryllium poisoning

Genetic Factors

Environmental Factors

Figure 11. Influence of environmental and genetic factors in atheroma development.

54

Summary

1 The arterial wall is a complex organ, constantly subjected to changes in blood composition and flow which may result in focal injury and subsequent repair.

2 In susceptible individuals, reparative processes may induce localized metabolic abnormalities and initiation of self-perpetuating arterial damage.

3 The organized atheromatous plaque is the multifaceted result of long-lasting, abnormal arterial wall metabolism and repair, slowly progressing toward overt clinical symptoms.

4 Current epidemiological and experimental studies suggest that by altering some primary risk factors the progression of some atherosclerotic lesions may be slowed or regression induced.

ACKNOWLEDGMENT

The following table and figure have been reproduced by permission of the authors and publishers.

Figure 5 and Table VII. Schettler G, Weizel A (eds): *International (III) Symposium on Atherosclerosis*, West Berlin, 1973. Courtesy of Springer-Verlag, New York, NY.

SECTION III

Diagnosis of Coronary Artery Disease

Stephen E. Epstein, MD

Chief, Cardiology Branch
National Heart and Lung Institute
National Institutes of Health
Bethesda, Maryland 20014

Note: This chapter was written by Dr. Epstein in his private
capacity. No official support or endorsement by the National
Institutes of Health or the Department of Health, Education,
and Welfare is intended or should be inferred.

The History

Over the past few decades, many sophisticated techniques have been developed to establish the diagnosis of coronary artery disease. Some of the techniques have been helpful, but others have served to confuse more than to enlighten. Some of the methods that the physician may use to determine whether or not his patient has coronary artery disease will be analyzed. Those particular diagnostic approaches are presented that, in the author's experience, either (1) have proven to be exceptionally valuable; (2) appear to hold great potential for the future but are still undergoing evaluation; or (3) are used very frequently, but often yield ambiguous information.

EVIDENCE OF ANGINA PECTORIS

One of the most reliable ways a physician can establish the diagnosis of functionally significant coronary artery disease is to determine whether or not the patient has angina pectoris. Such a diagnosis, however, is not as simple as many physicians believe, because many types of noncardiac chest discomfort often mimic angina pectoris. In order to establish definitively whether or not a given symptom complex indicates myocardial ischemia, the characteristics of the chest discomfort must be defined meticulously. Few better descriptions of characteristic features of angina pectoris can be found than Heberden's concise but eloquent account, first published in 1772:

They who are afflicted with it, are seized while they are walking (more especially if it be up hill, and soon after eating) with a painful and most disagreeable sensation in the breast, which seems as if it would extinguish life, if it were to increase or to continue; but the moment they stand still, all this uneasiness vanishes.

Angina pectoris has many patterns of presentation. It is most important for the student of cardiology to learn those attributes that are *essential* to diagnose angina with a high degree of certainty; then those features that *may* be present but are not necessarily components of the angina syndrome; and finally, those qualities of chest pain that do *not* suggest the diagnosis of angina pectoris (Tables I and II).

Quality: Angina pectoris often is not perceived by the patient as frank pain, but rather as deep, visceral distress described as a heavy, squeezing pressure or ache. This is an important distinction, since a patient with classic angina pectoris, if asked only whether or not he experiences chest *pain,* may deny its existence, leading the physician into a diagnostic error.

Location: The primary location and radiation of angina pectoris are described classically as substernal discomfort, radiating into the left shoulder and down the medial aspect of the left arm. The discomfort occasionally radiates to the right shoulder and arm, to the scapula, or to the neck, face, and jaw. Although radiation to one or more of these sites is commonly associated with the substernal discomfort, radiation of pain is not always present and is not necessary to establish the diagnosis of angina pectoris. However, if discomfort is experienced at these peripheral sites in the *absence* of a substernal component, the physician is not on very firm ground in making the diagnosis of angina.

Although some patients with myocardial ischemia will have pain *only* in these peripheral sites, noncardiac pain may also be experienced at similar sites, but will generally lack the characteristic substernal component of the true angina syndrome.

Duration: Typically, the duration of angina pectoris is almost invariably more than one minute and usually less than 15 minutes. Obviously, the discomfort of myocardial ischemia may be more prolonged when a patient has "crescendo" angina or if he is experiencing a frank myocardial infarction. However, if the *only* type of discomfort elicited by history lasts for longer than 15 minutes, it is most likely *not* caused by large-vessel coronary artery disease.

Precipitating factors: Many circumstances can precipitate or predispose the patient to an episode of angina pectoris. However, for a reliable diagnosis of coronary artery disease, the most important clue is precipitation of the discomfort by exercise. If exertion does not precipitate chest discomfort, the physician must be cautious in making the diagnosis of coronary artery disease. Patients who experience chest discomfort that is otherwise characteristic of angina pectoris, but is never brought on by exertion, often have no large-vessel coronary artery lesions.

Other characteristics: There are other characteristics of the angina syndrome that are helpful, but not necessary, in establishing the diagnosis of angina pectoris. The discomfort from angina is usually relieved by nitroglycerin. However, sublingual nitroglycerin takes about one to three minutes to act; therefore, the patient may not report relief with nitroglycerin if his discomfort disappears spontaneously in two or three minutes, as is often the case.

Another characteristic of angina is that the patient, in describing his discomfort, places his fist over his sternum. This

Table I.
Major characteristics of typical angina pectoris.

Deep visceral distress (heavy squeezing pressure or ache) experienced substernally

Onset occurs with exertion; relieved by rest

Duration: >1 min, <15 min

Features often associated with but not necessarily accompanying angina pectoris

Relief by nitroglycerin

Pain often described by placing fist on sternum (clenched-fist sign)

Pain precipitated by cold, emotion

More immediate relief in sitting or standing position than in supine position

Radiation to left shoulder and arm, or to neck and jaw

Table II.
Characteristics of chest pain suggesting a noncardiac origin.

Brief, rapid bursts of stabbing pain

Location in left side of chest or inframammary area

Duration <1 min or >20 min

Patient uses one finger to locate pain and to indicate size of area of involvement

Similar pain induced by pressing on chest wall

Pain altered by respiration

is the "clenched-fist" sign, a very reliable indicator of true angina pectoris.

It is also notable that angina is more apt to be precipitated when the patient exerts himself in cold weather. The circulatory changes responsible are partially due to vasoregulatory reflexes designed to maintain body temperature. These reflexes cause vasoconstriction and systemic arterial hypertension, thereby increasing myocardial oxygen consumption (see Section IV, MEDICAL TREATMENT OF STABLE ANGINA PECTORIS).

Another feature of angina pectoris is that the patient experiences more rapid symptomatic relief when sitting or standing. Patients usually avoid lying down when seeking relief from typical anginal discomfort, probably because of posturally induced alterations in myocardial oxygen consumption (MVO_2), ie, the left ventricle is larger when the patient is supine than when he is sitting or standing. This leads to a greater myocardial wall tension for any given intraventricular pressure, thereby increasing MVO_2.

CHARACTERISTICS SUGGESTING A DIAGNOSIS OF NONCARDIAC PAIN

Several kinds of chest discomfort suggest a noncardiac origin of the pain. Patients frequently describe having brief, rapid bursts of stabbing pain, or pain located in the left side of the chest or inframammary region. Such pains, with rare exception, can be disregarded as manifestations of coronary artery disease. The same is true of pain lasting less than one minute or more than 15 minutes. Although sometimes coronary artery discomfort does last for more than 15 minutes, if this is the *only* type of pain described, it is probably not due to large-vessel coronary disease.

Occasionally, a patient may use one finger to indicate the site of pain and the size of the involved area. Again, this is an unlikely sign of angina, since the deep visceral discomfort of true myocardial ischemia is rarely limited to a small area.

A frequent diagnostic error occurs when the physician ascribes pain originating in the chest wall to coronary artery disease. Angina pectoris is not altered by respiration. If the patient reports either worsening or relief of his discomfort with deep respiration, he may have pleurisy rather than angina. A search for chest-wall tenderness should be a routine part of the physician's examination. When pain that can be elicited by touch is identical to the pain experienced spontaneously, the discomfort most likely originates in the chest wall.

Referred pain, originating from cervical-nerve root disease, can also closely mimic the pain of myocardial ischemia. Such pain may occur at night in particular, leading to the diagnosis of nocturnal angina; it may be precipitated by exercise as well. The physician should be aware of these factors whenever a history of "angina" with atypical features is obtained. The correct diagnosis may be made by putting the patient through maneuvers that cause traction on the cervical nerves. If these maneuvers reproduce the chest discomfort, a noncardiac cause of the pain may be inferred. Of course, the demonstration of cervical disease does not rule out the existence of CAD.

CONCLUSION

If the chest discomfort is substernal, occurs with exertion, and is relieved by rest within several minutes, chances are very great that the discomfort is caused by coronary artery disease. If one of these features is not present, then the patient is having "atypical" chest discomfort, and the chances of coronary artery disease are considerably reduced. All of the other features of the discomfort provide ancillary clues; however, a reliable diagnosis of angina pectoris rests on substernal location, precipitation by exertion, and relief by rest.

EVIDENCE OF MYOCARDIAL INFARCTION

If myocardial infarction has been documented by typical ECG or enzyme changes, it is extremely likely that the patient has coronary artery disease. However, "classical" myocardial infarction has been described rarely in patients who were found to have normal coronary arteries. The cause of such infarction is doubtless the result of many factors. For example, we have found that it may occur in patients with severe myocardial hypertrophy due to hypertrophic cardiomyopathy (HCM); it may also be due to coronary emboli.

IMPORTANCE OF RISK FACTORS

The presence of such risk factors as hypercholesterolemia, high blood pressure, smoking, or family history of coronary artery disease tends to indicate a statistical probability that a patient will develop overt manifestations of coronary artery disease eventually. However, these factors are not helpful in determining whether coronary artery disease is actually present. Thus, the most important practical reason for obtaining information about risk factors is to determine possible therapeutic approaches that will reduce the likelihood of future complications.

Physical Examination

BASELINE EVALUATION

No single finding on physical examination contributes much to unequivocally establishing the diagnosis of coronary artery disease. Certain findings do, however, suggest either that a cardiac abnormality is present or that the patient is at greater risk of developing overt manifestations of coronary artery disease. For example, although the presence of an S4 on auscultation is compatible with coronary artery disease, it is a nonspecific finding also present in patients with hypertension, HCM, or aortic stenosis. Further, an apical midsystolic or holosystolic murmur may indicate papillary muscle dysfunction due to coronary artery disease. As an isolated finding, however, it is more likely indicative of abnormalities other than coronary artery disease; for example, rheumatic heart disease, mitral valve prolapse, or HCM. Occasionally, an anterior systolic bulge indicative of a left ventricular aneurysm can be palpated. But, since this is such an uncommon finding, it rarely aids in diagnosing coronary artery disease.

There are other findings on physical examination that place a patient in a higher risk category for developing coronary artery disease, but these in themselves do not help to diagnose existing disease. They include (1) an *arcus senilis* in patients less than 50 years of age; (2) xanthomas typical of type II, III, or IV hyperlipoproteinemia (as described in Section I), as well as (3) hypertension.

EVALUATION DURING AN EPISODE OF ANGINA

If the physician happens to be examining a patient during an episode of angina, the following changes suggest coronary artery disease: (1) the development of a late systolic murmur (indicative of papillary muscle dysfunction); (2) the development of an S4; and (3) the relief of pain by carotid sinus massage (Levine sign). Carotid sinus massage abolishes angina mainly because of baroreceptor-mediated reflexes that lead to bradycardia and lowering of systemic arterial pressure, both of which reduce MVO_2 and thereby reestablish the balance between myocardial oxygen supply and demand. The massage technique can be of considerable help, but it must be applied with caution in older patients or in those suspected of having cerebrovascular disease.

The Electrocardiogram

BASELINE ECG

The baseline ECG in a patient with coronary artery disease is very often normal; therefore, the ECG is an insensitive marker of coronary artery disease. When the ECG is abnormal, the most specific findings indicative of coronary artery disease are Q waves occurring in the characteristic patterns of inferior wall infarction (Q waves in leads II and III, and AVF) or anterolateral wall infarction (Q waves in lead I and AVL). It must be emphasized, however, that although such abnormal Q wave patterns were at one time considered pathognomonic of myocardial infarction due to coronary artery disease, "infarct" patterns indistinguishable from those associated with coronary disease are now known to occur commonly in patients with HCM (Figure 1). Coronary artery disease can also cause T-wave inversions and ST-segment depressions unassociated with QRS abnormalities, but these findings occur under many conditions and are, therefore, highly nonspecific. On the other hand, ST-segment elevation suggests myocardial scar or aneurysm secondary to coronary artery disease.

ECG DURING AN EPISODE OF ANGINA

Changes in ECG patterns recorded during an episode of chest pain (typical of that the patient presented with) may help in establishing the diagnosis of coronary artery disease. Thus, severe coronary artery disease is usually present if frank ST-segment elevation develops during chest discomfort (Prinzmetal angina, Figure 2). However, some patients with Prinzmetal-type angina have essentially normal coronary arteries. In some of these patients it now has been established that the chest discomfort and ST-segment elevations are associated with coronary artery spasm. The development of ST-segment depression and T-wave inversion during a spontaneous attack of chest pain also suggests the presence of coronary artery disease. However, it, too, can be caused by coronary spasm.

ECG EXERCISE TESTING

Although acute changes occur in the ECG during spontaneous attacks of angina pectoris while the patient is at rest, similar reversible changes can be precipitated during episodes of angina pectoris induced by exercise. These findings led to the suspicion that exercise-induced ECG changes, even in the absence of angina pectoris, were indicative of myocardial ischemia. For the past 40 years, therefore, analysis of the ECG response to exercise has been favored as a simple noninvasive aid in the diagnosis of ischemic heart disease.

Figure 1. Deep, wide Q waves are present in leads I, AVL, V5, and V6. ST-segment elevation also is present in these leads. This electrocardiogram is compatible with either acute anterolateral myocardial infarction or old anterolateral myocardial infarction with associated anterolateral aneurysm.

Electrocardiogram of a patient with hypertrophic cardiomyopathy

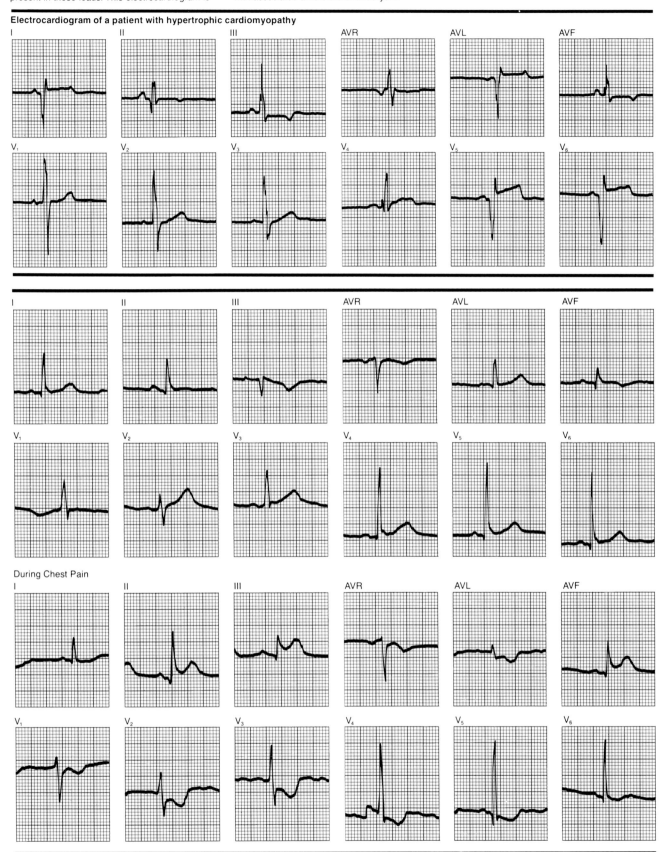

Figure 2. ECG demonstrating changes associated with Prinzmetal angina. Pronounced ST-segment elevation develops in leads II, III, AVF, and a marked shift in the T-wave vector occurs during a spontaneous episode of chest pain. (Courtesy of Robert A. O'Rourke, MD.)

Considerable advances have been made in the techniques for administering an exercise test. These include (1) the development of improved electrodes; (2) an awareness of the necessity for good skin-electrode preparation; and (3) the importance of observing changes in the ECG during, as well as immediately after, exercise.

Considerable attention has also been directed to the criteria used to determine if test findings are normal or abnormal. It now is generally accepted that only ST-segment changes should be employed in this determination. To minimize the possibility of false-positive results, an exercise ECG is consid-

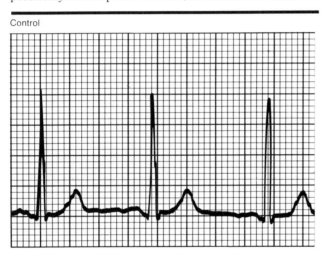

Control

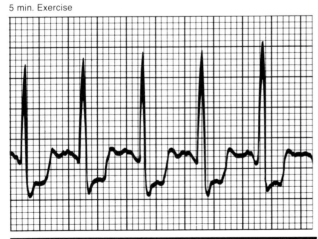

5 min. Exercise

Figure 3. Typical example of a markedly positive ECG response to exercise. This patient, with severe occlusive disease of the left anterior descending, circumflex, and right coronary arteries, developed pronounced ST-segment depression during exercise but experienced no chest discomfort during the test. (Courtesy of Robert A. O'Rourke, MD.)

ered positive by most investigators only if, 0.08 seconds after the J point, the ST segment is depressed at least 0.1 mV below the resting baseline value, with the slope of that segment ≤ 0 (Figure 3). Using these or similar criteria, numerous epidemiologic studies of large groups of subjects have documented the value of exercise electrocardiography in predicting the likelihood of subsequent manifestations of myocardial ischemia (angina pectoris, myocardial infarction, or coronary death).

LIMITATIONS OF EXERCISE TESTING

A test that predicts the statistical likelihood that disease is present in a subgroup of a large number of subjects is not necessarily an accurate predictor of disease in a specific patient. Thus, when the same test used in epidemiologic studies is used to diagnose coronary disease in the patient, it is critical to know how often a "positive" response indicates underlying coronary artery disease and how often it is a "false-positive" result. Likewise, it is important to know how often a "negative" response defines the absence of disease, and how often it is a "false-negative" result.

Before examining these questions, let us define our terms. Conventionally, the sensitivity of a test is defined as the percentage of patients with known disease who have a positive response:

$$\left(\frac{\text{true positive}}{\text{true positive} + \text{false negative}}\right)$$

The specificity of a test is defined as measuring the likelihood that a patient known to be free of disease will have a negative exercise test:

$$\left(\frac{\text{true negative}}{\text{true negative} + \text{false positive}}\right)$$

Finally, the predictive value of a test is defined as the likelihood that an individual with a given test result does or does not have disease:

$$\left(\frac{\text{true negative}}{\text{true negative} + \text{false negative}}\right) \quad \left(\frac{\text{true positive}}{\text{true positive} + \text{false positive}}\right)$$

The key to understanding the limitations of ECG exercise testing is the fact that the sensitivity and predictive value of the test are critically dependent upon the nature of the population under study. For example, it is commonly believed that the sensitivity of ECG exercise testing is well over 90%. However, recent studies demonstrate that sensitivity varies according to the extent and severity of the coronary artery disease. Thus, a higher percentage of positive exercise tests occurs in patients with triple-vessel disease than in patients with single- or double-vessel disease. Also, where the same number of diseased vessels exists, a higher percentage of positive results occurs in patients with greater than 75% coronary artery narrowing than in those with 50% to 75% narrowing.

Given these results, it is obvious that a very high test sensitivity will be reported by laboratories to which severely symptomatic patients are referred for coronary artery surgery, since such patients tend to have severe coronary disease. Conversely, the practicing physician should anticipate a much lower test sensitivity, since he generally sees patients with less severe symptoms and presumably less severe coronary disease. The results of a recent National Institutes of Health (NIH) study illustrate this point. Patients with hypercholesterolemia were included in the study, but those with symptoms severe enough to warrant operative intervention were excluded. Of the patients in the study who had previous myocardial infarction, typical angina pectoris, or both, approximately *two thirds* had *negative* exercise tests. Moreover, the highest percentage of coronary patients with a positive exercise test were those who had greater than 75% coronary artery narrowing and significant disease involving all three major coronary arteries. Even in this group, however, the frequency of false-negative responses was over 35%.

Specificity is defined by statisticians as the measure of the likelihood that a patient known to be free of coronary disease will have a negative test. It is of limited applicability in the clinical situation where the relevant statistic is the likelihood that either (1) an individual having coronary disease will have a negative test, or (2) an individual with a positive exercise test will have coronary disease (ie, predictive value). As with sensitivity, it had been assumed (from studies performed in highly selected patient populations) that the predictive value of the ECG response to exercise in establishing the diagnosis of coronary artery disease was very high.

It is a mathematically demonstrable fact that the lower the prevalence of a disease in a study population, the greater the likelihood that a positive test will be falsely positive (Table III, Figure 4). This is best appreciated by studying the simple calculations illustrated in Table III, in which it has been assumed that exercise testing has a sensitivity $\left(\frac{TP}{TP + FN}\right)$ and specificity $\left(\frac{TN}{TN + FP}\right)$ of 95%. The upper panel of Table III displays the calculations in a patient population in which coronary artery disease is present in 90% of the patients (such as might be found in an institution to which patients with

Figure 4. Influence of disease prevalence on predictive accuracy of a positive exercise test. The curve was generated by employing the mathematical techniques described in the text. It was assumed that the exercise test was 95% sensitive and 95% specific. Change in sensitivity has little effect on the curve. A decrease in specificity, however, shifts the curve to the right, which would lower predictive accuracy for any given disease prevalence. This figure indicates that if a population of subjects with a 2% disease prevalence were studied, a positive ECG response to exercise would have a predictive accuracy of only about 25%. If disease prevalence were greater than 50%, however, predictive accuracy would be 95% or better.

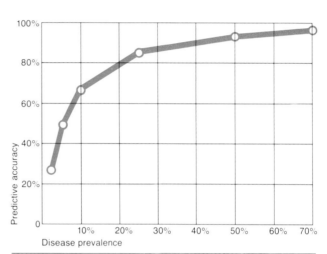

Assumption: Test is 95% sensitive and 95% specific.

Table III.
Influence of disease prevalence on predictive accuracy of a positive exercise test.

Disease prevalence = 90%
Test 95% sensitive and 95% specific

Subjects	Number with positive test	Number with negative test
900 diseased	855	45
100 nondiseased	5	95
TOTAL 1000	860	140

Predictive accuracy $= \frac{855}{860} = 99\%$

Disease prevalence = 2%
Test 95% sensitive and 95% specific

Subjects	Number with positive test	Number with negative test
20 diseased	19	1
980 nondiseased	49	931
TOTAL 1000	68	932

Predictive accuracy $= \frac{19}{68} = 28\%$

severe symptoms of coronary artery disease are referred for possible operative intervention). The lower panel of Table III displays calculations based on a population of subjects with a disease prevalence of only 2% (such as might exist in an otherwise unselected group of individuals free of any signs or symptoms of coronary disease, ie, those individuals subjected to a "routine" ECG exercise test during an annual physical examination).

The different values for predictive accuracy in the two populations derives from the large differences in the number of normal subjects and, hence, from the large differences in the *absolute* number of subjects who will have false-positive results, assuming that the test yields 5% false-positive results (95% specific). Thus, although the percentage of subjects in the population with low disease prevalence who have a false-positive test is small, the absolute number of such patients, derived from the relatively large group of non-diseased subjects, will be much higher than the number of true-positive results derived from the relatively small group of diseased subjects. The influence of disease prevalence in the population being studied (on the predictive accuracy of a positive test) is depicted graphically in Figure 4. This graph illustrates that predictive accuracy decreases precipitously after disease prevalence falls below 25%.

Thus, the explanation for the high predictive value of a positive exercise test found in most published series undoubtedly is that the study populations were confined largely to patients with angina pectoris or previous myocardial infarction (a population with a high CAD prevalence). In contrast, the studies reporting low predictive value of ECG exercise tests were based on results derived from asymptomatic populations (populations expected to have a low CAD prevalence).

EVALUATION OF EXERCISE TESTING

A patient with a negative ECG response to exercise is far more likely than a patient with a positive test to have normal coronary arteries and to remain free of the manifestations of coronary disease over the next several years. Some studies suggest that over 15 times the number of patients with a positive ECG response to exercise go on to develop overt manifestations of coronary disease, compared to the number with a negative ECG response who develop manifestations of CAD (Table III). This point is of epidemiologic importance.

However, different criteria must be used to determine whether a test is helpful for the individual patient. It is clear that, when a patient has a history of classic angina pectoris or a well-documented history of previous myocardial infarction, the history is more accurate than an exercise test in establishing the existence of coronary artery disease. In such cases, ECG exercise testing is of dubious value as a diagnostic tool. At the opposite extreme are individuals who have no cardiac symptoms. Exercise ECG tests performed routinely in this population undoubtedly result in much more harm than good. The large number of false-positive tests that would necessarily occur might cause psychological and economic problems in many normal, disease-free subjects.

By employing more rigid ECG criteria for ischemia, it is possible to enhance predictive accuracy. Thus, if ST-segment depression of ≥ 2 mm is present during exercise, specificity will increase, and the curve depicted in Figure 4 will be shifted to the left, thereby increasing the predictive value of a positive test for any patient population studied. However, as is apparent from Figure 4, this will not eliminate the possibility that an occasional patient who shows pronounced ST-segment depression has no significant disease detectable by angiography.

On the other hand, the test may be of greater utility in patients with atypical chest pain. Disease prevalence is relatively high in such a population; thus, the predictive accuracy of an exercise test in this situation should be relatively good (Figure 4).

The advantage of employing rigid criteria is that false-positive diagnoses of coronary artery disease will decrease. However, the disadvantage of such rigid criteria is that the test becomes extremely insensitive, because the majority of patients with documented coronary disease will not develop such pronounced ST-segment depression. In fact, it has been shown that over 50% of symptomatic patients with left main- or triple-vessel disease have either normal ST-segment response to exercise or develop depression of less than 2 mm.

Despite the limitations of the ECG response to exercise in diagnosing coronary artery disease, it must be emphasized that other uses of exercise testing are of great value. For example, if substernal chest discomfort develops during exercise and is relieved after a few minutes of rest, a reliable diagnosis of coronary disease can be made in a patient with an equivocal history of chest pain. Moreover, the patient's exercise capacity can be objectively ascertained, and it can be determined whether or not exercise precipitates serious ventricular arrhythmias.

Radiographic Techniques

CHEST RADIOGRAPHY

Routine chest radiography is not very helpful in diagnosing coronary artery disease. Usually, the patient with angina pectoris due to coronary artery disease has a normal-sized heart with no evidence of pulmonary venous congestion. Even patients with dilated left ventricles on left ventricular angiography will often have normal chest x-ray findings. When severe left ventricular failure is present, the heart on x-ray may appear dilated, with evidence of pulmonary venous hypertension, but these findings are not specific for coronary disease. Occasionally, a frank aneurysmal bulge can be seen along the left cardiac border, a finding highly suggestive of CAD. However, most aneurysms demonstrated by ventriculography are either not evident on x-ray or give only the appearance of a dilated heart.

CARDIAC FLUOROSCOPY

In contrast, fluoroscopic examination of the heart for detection of coronary artery calcifications can be helpful. Thus, an NIH study of hypercholesterolemic patients revealed that if coronary calcifications were observed in an asymptomatic subject less than 55 years of age, there was a better-than-90% chance that some degree of coronary arterial narrowing, demonstrated by angiography, was present. About one third of all the patients, however, had coronary artery narrowing of less than 50%. They might, therefore, be considered to fall into the false-positive group, at least with regard to the presence of a significantly narrowed coronary artery. Hence, the predictive accuracy of this test for detecting functionally significant coronary narrowing in asymptomatic subjects with hypercholesterolemia is approximately 55%.

It is important to emphasize that an experienced radiologist must carry out this examination. Small amounts of calcium may be missed by the untutored eye, and valvular or pericardial calcification can be misinterpreted as representing coronary artery calcification. Nevertheless, even when an experienced radiologist performs the examinations, a large number of patients with underlying coronary artery disease (about 55% of the population referred to above) show no visible calcifications at fluoroscopy. Hence, this screening test is not very sensitive.

ECHOCARDIOGRAPHY

Echocardiography is most helpful in ruling out entities that may closely simulate coronary artery disease, in terms of its

Figure 5. The ventricular septum is massively thickened, whereas the posterior wall is only moderately so. The position and motion of the mitral valve also demonstrate findings characteristic of HCM: the valve is positioned more anteriorly at onset of systole; diastolic closing slope is slow; and there is abnormal anterior systolic motion of the mitral leaflets.

Echocardiogram of a patient with hypertrophic cardiomyopathy.

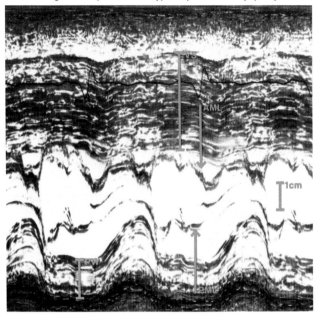

VS: ventricular septum   PW: posterior wall
AML: anterior mitral valve leaflet   PML: posterior mitral valve leaflet

symptomatic or electrocardiographic presentation. For example, a patient with hypertrophic cardiomyopathy (HCM) is often brought to the physician's attention because of a history of chest discomfort. Characteristically, the pain is not as predictably related to exertion as is the pain caused by coronary artery disease. It usually lasts longer and may be relieved, rather than exacerbated, by a cold environment. Nonetheless, many patients with HCM have classic angina pectoris and frequently have prominent ECG abnormalities, including Q wave patterns "diagnostic" of CAD (Figure 1). The echocardiographic examination, by demonstrating the disproportionately thickened ventricular septum (Figure 5) can establish the diagnosis of HCM (which, of course, does not rule out the possibility of coexisting coronary artery disease). Similarly, patients with mitral valve prolapse often have atypical chest pain, sometimes associated with atrial or ventricular arrhythmias. ST-T wave abnormalities on the ECG are also common. Echocardiographic evaluation of the patient will alert the physician to the presence of mitral valve prolapse, even when the typical auscultatory findings of prolapse are ambiguous or absent (Figure 6).

64

Echocardiogram of a patient with mitral valve prolapse.

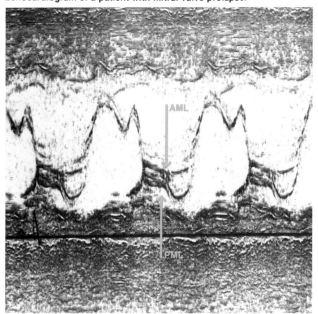

AML: anterior mitral valve leaflet
PML: posterior mitral valve leaflet

Figure 6. During mid-systole, the posterior leaflet of the mitral valve moves abruptly away from the sternum.

LIMITATIONS OF ECHOCARDIOGRAPHY

Echocardiography is of great value in detecting diseases that may mimic some features of coronary artery disease; however, it is not very helpful in establishing the diagnosis of CAD. The major limitation of echocardiography in diagnosing coronary artery disease is its restricted resolution capacity, which prevents visualization of the coronary arteries. However, functional consequences of the underlying disorder sometimes can be detected, which leads to the suspicion of coronary disease. Thus, patients with left anterior descending coronary disease may demonstrate abnormal (paradoxical) movement of the ventricular septum: during systole, the septum moves anteriorly toward the sternum rather than posteriorly away from the sternum.

Similarly, although some patients with left anterior descending coronary disease demonstrate a normal pattern of movement, the magnitude of systolic movement is reduced in relation to systolic motion of the posterior left ventricular wall.

The opposite finding can occasionally be observed in patients with disease of the vessels that supply the posterobasal left ventricular wall. Although such observations should raise the possibility of underlying coronary disease, abnormal septal motion is found in patients with conduction abnormalities (such as left-bundle branch block, or Wolff-Parkinson-White syndrome), and in patients with any disorder producing right ventricular dilatation (such as left-to-right shunts or right ventricular hypertension). Finally, if septal thickness is less than posterior wall thickness by 2 mm or more, old septal infarction with septal atrophy should be suspected.

Another limitation of echocardiography is that the echo beam cannot traverse bony structures and the lung, confining echo "visualization" of the heart to the ventricular septum and posterior left ventricular wall. This limitation is not of great practical importance in studying diseases that cause diffuse abnormalities of myocardial function. In coronary artery disease, however, the limitation is crucial, since the functional abnormalities are segmental. Thus, severe abnormalities of myocardial contractile function, involving the anterior, anterolateral, or apical portions of the left ventricle, cannot be detected directly by routine echocardiographic examination. Techniques to circumvent this limitation are being evaluated, but in all likelihood, the major contribution of conventional one-dimensional echocardiography will be to rule out diseases that may simulate some of the features of coronary artery disease.

Another approach that may be much more helpful in evaluating CAD patients is sector-scanning (two-dimensional) echocardiography. This newly emerging technique allows a pie-shaped section of the heart to be scanned in real time so that a better visualization of segmental disorders of contraction can be obtained (Figure 7). Some preliminary work even suggests that the left and right coronary arteries, at their origin, can be imaged by this technique. Several years of research will be necessary, however, before the scope and usefulness of this more sophisticated method of echocardiography can be assessed.

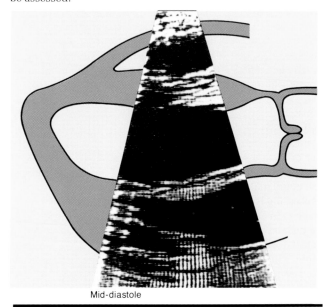

Mid-diastole

Figure 7. Sector-scan (two-dimensional echocardiogram) of a normal subject. The echo transducer is very rapidly rotated mechanically over a 30° sector, producing a two-dimensional sagittal image of the heart.

Cardiac Catheterization

CORONARY ANGIOGRAPHY

One of the most important advances in diagnostic cardiology over the past two decades has been the development of angiographic techniques permitting adequate visualization of coronary vessels as small as 0.5 mm in diameter. Thus, by selective injection of contrast material into the coronary arteries, the patency of the large coronary arteries as well as the presence of coronary collaterals can be assessed (Figures 8A, 8B). This development has been the most outstanding stimulus to the application of surgical approaches to the treatment of coronary disease.

Conversely, the success of coronary artery bypass surgery in the treatment of a patient with severe angina has made essential the precise anatomic definition and localization of lesions obstructing the large coronary arteries. Further, determination of the number of diseased coronary arteries helps predict whether the patient is in a high-risk or a low-risk group. Such information influences the ultimate decision whether or not to perform coronary bypass.

Because coronary angiography provides the physician with such an extraordinarily powerful diagnostic tool, the problems and limitations inherent in this technique must be completely understood. First, there are risks associated with the procedure. The magnitude of these risks is related to the experience and skills of the coronary angiographer. In a good laboratory, with senior physicians performing the study, the risk to life should be less than one per 1,000 studies. Similar risks exist for nonfatal coronary artery dissection with resultant myocardial infarction, as well as for nonfatal embolic complications arising from clots forming on the tip of the catheter. (Such clots can embolize either to the distal coronary tree, with resultant acute myocardial infarction, or to the cerebral vessels, with resultant stroke.)

Second, accurate anatomic information depends on a number of factors, including the skills of the angiographer performing the catheterization, the skills of the physician reading the angiograms, and the quality of the equipment and film-processing techniques. Even if all of these factors are optimal, there is the distinct possibility that a high-grade lesion may be dismissed as insignificant or may go undetected. Studies correlating coronary artery narrowing assessed by angiography with that found at necropsy have demonstrated that the severity of disease is frequently underestimated at angiography. In addition, a total occlusion or high-grade lesion at the origin of a branch of one of the major coronary arteries may not be detected, particularly when a plethora of overlapping vessels does not allow the angiographer to see each vessel as a separate entity. This latter problem has been minimized by obtaining multiple views of the vessels in addition to the standard lateral and oblique projections.

One additional limitation of coronary angiography needs mention: the technique is used as the standard for determining the presence of ischemic disease. However, it is possible that myocardial ischemia, a physiologic abnormality, may exist in the absence of angiographically demonstrable large-vessel disease, an anatomic abnormality. In particular, the resolution capabilities of currently available equipment are such that the physician cannot make the diagnosis of "small-vessel coronary disease," an entity that has recently received increased attention. However, while this is a diagnostic limitation of coronary angiography, from a therapeutic point of view (as regards application of coronary bypass surgery) the most important information the physician needs is whether or not large-vessel coronary disease is present.

LEFT VENTRICULAR ANGIOGRAPHY

Left ventricular cineangiography is an integral part of the catheterization assessment of a patient with coronary disease. This is traditionally performed in most laboratories in the right anterior oblique position, thereby permitting visualization of the silhouette of the diaphragmatic, anterior, and apical portions of the left ventricle. This view, however, does not permit assessment of contractile function of the septal, anterolateral, and posterior portions of the left ventricle — information that can be obtained if the ventriculogram is also assessed in the left anterior oblique position. Using one or, preferably, both projections, a rough estimate of overall ventricular function can be made, as well as more precise estimates of the severity of segmental abnormalities of myocardial function. This information, along with that provided by coronary angiography, helps define the patient's prognostic subgroup. It also helps establish the risks to the patient if he undergoes a coronary bypass operation. (The risks are considerably higher for the patient with a large, dilated left ventricle, or one with a substantial portion of myocardium that is contracting poorly.)

Recent studies suggest that important information might be obtained by performing left ventricular cineangiographic studies before and after the administration of nitroglycerin. Thus, an improvement in systolic motion of the myocardium

Figure 8A. Angiogram of the left coronary system in a normal subject, right anterior oblique (RAO) position.

LMCA: left main coronary artery
CIRC: circumflex coronary artery
LAD: left anterior descending coronary artery

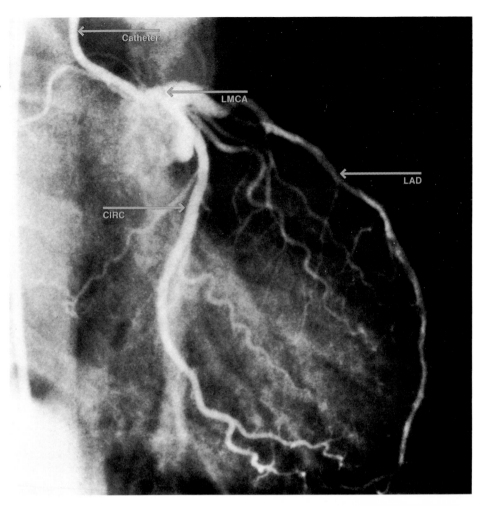

Figure 8B. Angiogram of the left coronary system of a patient with severe coronary artery disease.

The heavy arrows point to areas of major narrowing within the left anterior descending (LAD) and circumflex (CIRC) coronary arteries. Severe obstruction of the right coronary artery is also evident, as the distal right system fills retrogradely to the point of total occlusion (heavy arrow) via extensive collaterals from the circumflex and LAD systems (RAO position).

CIRC: circumflex coronary artery
LAD: left anterior descending coronary artery
LMCA: left main coronary artery
OM: oblique marginal coronary artery
RCA: right coronary artery

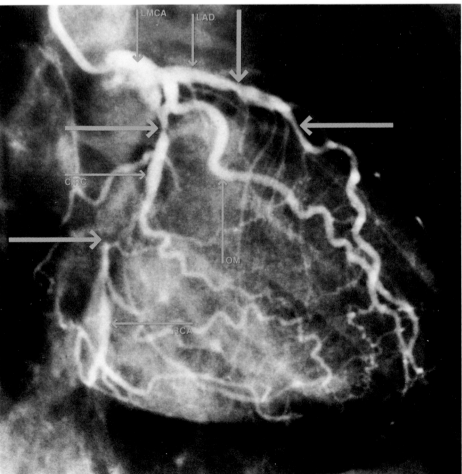

Radionuclides in the Diagnosis of Coronary Artery Disease

over baseline conditions can occur following nitroglycerin administration, an effect possibly caused by decreased ventricular afterload, increased myocardial perfusion, or both. Conversion of an akinetic or dyskinetic pattern of motion to hypokinetic or normal motion implies that a given portion of the left ventricle, instead of consisting of scar tissue, contains hypoperfused but viable myocardium. Therefore, the ventricle is potentially salvageable by coronary artery bypass operation. This information may eventually prove to be of great help in determining surgical approaches to the patient with coronary disease, but more research is necessary.

OTHER TESTS PERFORMED AT CATHETERIZATION
Another approach used in the catheterization laboratory is to assess whether the myocardium is consuming or producing lactate. This is determined by measuring arteriovenous difference of lactate across the coronary bed, often before and after a standard stress procedure, such as increasing heart rate by atrial pacing. Measuring lactate has great theoretical value in determining whether the myocardium has changed from aerobic to anaerobic pathways of metabolism. So far, however, the practical utility of this test has not been very great. This may be, in part, because coronary artery disease is a segmental abnormality, and sampling coronary venous blood from the coronary sinus produces a mixed sample of lactate derived from large portions of the left ventricle. Whether or not modification of this technique will result in greater usefulness remains to be determined.

Myocardial and blood-pool imaging techniques provide information not obtainable with coronary angiography. For example, these techniques can (1) determine whether equivocally significant anatomic abnormalities, defined by angiography, produce functionally significant impairment in myocardial perfusion; (2) delineate the site of an infarction, which then may eventually provide a quantitative measure of the extent of myocardial necrosis; and (3) image the intraventricular blood pool, thereby providing a noninvasive alternative to angiography for determining overall ventricular function as well as detecting areas of segmental dysfunction.

Several types of studies are currently being carried out with radiopharmaceuticals to provide the cardiologist with this information. Some of these studies involve the following:
Detection of Myocardial Perfusion Defects
The radionuclides commonly employed in such studies are potassium-42, potassium-43, and thallium-201; as well as macroaggregates of albumin labeled with ^{131}I or ^{99m}Tc, and human albumin microspheres usually labeled with ^{99m}Tc.
Detection of Acute Myocardial Infarction
Radionuclides most commonly used at present include pyrophosphate, polyphosphate, or glucoheptinate, each labeled with ^{99m}Tc.
Assessment of Overall and Regional Myocardial Contractility
The most commonly used tracers for these studies are human serum albumin or red blood cells labeled with ^{99m}Tc.

MYOCARDIAL PERFUSION DEFECTS
Radioactive potassium and its analogs are taken up by normal ventricular myocardium. The resulting myocardial radioactivity can be imaged. In the presence of acute myocardial ischemia or infarction, zones of decreased or absent radioactivity (cold spots) occur. Similar results are obtained with radionuclides of cesium and thallium. Myocardial uptake of these agents depends on (1) the rate of delivery of these agents, which in turn is a function of myocardial blood flow; (2) the integrity of intracellular ion-concentrating mechanisms; and (3) the integrity of cell membranes. A deficiency of any of these mechanisms impairs the capacity of the myocardium to concentrate these isotopes, which produces a myocardial image containing diminished radioactivity. Such a cold spot may be indicative of (1) myocardial scar with diminished myocardial cellular mass and flow; (2) an absolute reduction in blood flow to myocardial tissue; or (3) a relative

inadequacy of myocardial flow, such as might occur during exercise or pacing-induced angina. Myocardial ischemia present under the latter two conditions may contribute to the defect in radionuclide concentration.

Potassium or, more recently, thallium-201 has been injected intravenously to determine if there are regional abnormalities of flow distribution in patients suspected of having coronary artery disease. In the absence of myocardial scar, patients with coronary artery disease and angina pectoris often have homogeneous distribution of the tracer under resting conditions. This would indicate that, despite coronary artery narrowing, flow to potentially ischemic regions is normal under baseline conditions. During exercise, however, coronary blood flow increases substantially in response to augmented myocardial oxygen requirements. The mechanism leading to increased coronary flow is impaired when high-grade proximal lesions are present. Although the amount of radionuclide distributed to myocardial capillary beds may be relatively uniform under the low-flow conditions present at rest, the disparity in flow to regions supplied by normal and abnormal coronary arteries during intense exercise would result in nonhomogeneous uptake of radionuclide. In addition, ischemia causes impairment of cell membrane function, which maintains transmembrane gradients of potassium or thallium, further interfering with radionuclide uptake in the ischemic bed.

These observations suggest that such an approach may be potentially useful as a screening test for coronary disease. However, as with the ST-segment response to exercise, the sensitivity and predictive accuracy of this technique must be determined before conclusions can be reached as to the utility of myocardial imaging.

ENHANCING THE IMAGE

One limitation inherent in the preceding techniques, using intravenous administration of tracer, is the inability to discriminate small areas of ischemia, or reduced flow. Resolution is enhanced, however, by imaging the myocardium through direct intracoronary administration of radioactive tracers. In practice, this technique requires injection of small labeled particles into the coronary arteries. The particles remain within the vessels, embolizing to and lodging within the distal coronary vessels. Particle distribution is related to coronary flow patterns. Although this technique requires the use of microemboli to delineate flow patterns, it appears to be safe and without measurable deleterious effect on myocardial function.

Particles currently employed are macroaggregates of albumin labeled with ^{131}I, and human albumin microspheres labeled with ^{131}Tc. The resulting myocardial images, when analyzed in conjunction with routine coronary angiography, can, in some patients, provide important information. Injection of the particles causes homogeneous distribution of radioactivity in patients with normal coronary arteries or with lesions that do not result in inadequate perfusion under resting conditions. In contrast, patients with myocardial scars or with functionally significant obstructions will show areas of diminished radioactivity.

Moreover, when a lesion of equivocal severity is associated with a normal myocardial image under baseline conditions, a second tracer can be injected during pacing-induced stress. Such studies, analogous to the exercise scintigraphic techniques using intravenously administered potassium or thallium, show that nonhomogeneous particle distribution may occur during pacing in individuals who had normal studies under baseline conditions (Figure 9). This technique is particularly valuable in the patient with chest discomfort whose coronary arterial narrowing observed on coronary angiography is estimated to be less than 50%, ie, "functionally insignificant." The anatomic severity of a lesion is occasionally underestimated by coronary angiography.

Myocardial imaging during pacing or exercise can help determine whether or not regional perfusion is adequate when the demand for myocardial blood flow is increased – the setting in which angina usually occurs in the patient with symptomatic coronary disease.

Even though the intracoronary injection of radionuclides appears to hold great promise for further defining abnormalities in myocardial perfusion, the technique presents some potential problems of unknown significance. For example, it is uncertain whether the particles mix adequately with blood when they are injected directly into a vessel as small as a coronary artery. If mixing is inadequate, particle distribution may be appreciably affected by blood-flow streaming, resulting in nonhomogeneous areas of radioactivity, even without a functionally significant defect in myocardial perfusion. Such a problem does not occur with intravenous injections of thallium or potassium, because there is ample opportunity for the tracer to mix with the blood. On the other hand, definition of defects is considerably enhanced by intra-

Figure 9. Under control conditions (top panel), the first radioisotope injection demonstrated homogenous perfusion of the left ventricle. When heart rate was increased by atrial pacing (bottom panel), a second isotope was injected.

Anterior and apical walls of the left ventricle show an area of relatively poor perfusion.

The patient had severe narrowing of the left anterior descending coronary artery.

Double-isotope technique for demonstrating areas of impaired perfusion.

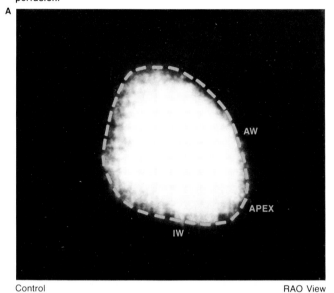

A

Control   RAO View

B

Pacing   RAO View

AW: anterior wall
IW: inferior wall

---

coronary injection of tracers.

Experience with myocardial imaging, obtained by either intravenous or intracoronary administration of radioisotope tracer, is still limited; thus, the precise role of each in the diagnostic armory of the physician remains to be explained.

DETECTION OF ACUTE MYOCARDIAL INFARCTION

When extracted by normal myocardium, radiopharmaceuticals such as potassium and thallium outline areas of acutely infarcted tissue. However, these tracers do not permit differentiation of myocardium undergoing acute necrosis (acute myocardial infarction) from fibrotic or previously infarcted tissue, or from myocardium undergoing transient and reversible ischemia. Ideally, isotopic delineation of acute myocardial infarction should be accomplished with a radiopharmaceutical that is selectively incorporated by irreversibly damaged myocardium. Such an agent would appear as a "hot spot," which would be more readily detectable than the "cold spot" produced by potassium or thallium.

Several such imaging agents have been used that seem to adequately delineate an area of acute necrosis. The agents that have received the most attention are ^{99m}Tc-labeled tetracycline, pyrophosphate, diphosphate, polyphosphate, and glucoheptinate. Tetracycline seems to bind to denatured protein and nucleic acids. It has been suggested that calcium may play an indirect role in binding tetracycline to these substances. Pyrophosphate is believed to be precipitated by calcium aggregates present in damaged mitochondria.

In studies employing labeled tetracycline, the drug has been found to be taken up preferentially by infarcted tissue within a few hours after infarction. Maximal concentration in infarcted tissue, as compared to normal tissue, occurs at about 24 hours. Scanning is complicated, however, because the drug "labels" the liver, making identification of diaphragmatic wall infarctions somewhat difficult. Moreover, an additional interval of 24 hours after injection of labeled tetracycline is necessary for optimal imaging of the infarct, because of the prolonged presence of high levels of the radionuclide in the bloodstream. ^{99m}Tc-labeled pyrophosphate appears to have certain advantages over tetracycline, eg, pyrophosphate images necrosing myocardium earlier after infarction, and it does not label the liver. Imaging, then, can be started earlier after injection of the tracer.

Several studies that involved the use of labeled tetracycline, pyrophosphate, and similar agents to delineate an acute infarct have yielded somewhat divergent results. Some investigators report an extraordinarily high reliability of the technique, with few false positives and false negatives. Other investigators emphasize that, although large transmural myocardial infarctions are easy to identify, difficulty occurs with smaller transmural or subendocardial infarctions. Estimates of false-positive and false-negative diagnoses using these radionuclides have ranged as high as 20%.

However, critical assessment of what constitutes a false-positive test is difficult. If a myocardial scan is positive and the diagnosis of myocardial infarction is made, but the patient has neither elevation of enzymes nor diagnostic changes on the ECG, is the scan "false positive" or is it more sensitive than serum enzymes or the ECG for diagnosing acute infarction?

Problems also arise regarding optimal time for radionuclide injection. Administration of the tracer either too soon or too late may lead to false-negative diagnoses. Serial injections of some isotopes may be difficult because of their relatively long half-life. Finally, it is still not clear to what extent reversible ischemia may also cause accumulation of labeled radioisotopes.

USE OF POSITRON EMITTERS
In addition to these commonly used radiopharmaceuticals, positron emitters, such as ^{13}N, have also been used for imaging infarcts. Since the half-life of ^{13}N is very short (less than ten minutes), serial studies become feasible. When combined with sophisticated computer technology, very high-quality images of ischemic portions of myocardium have been defined with positron emitters (Figure 10). However, because of the extremely short half-life of these isotopes, they, of necessity, can be used only in facilities equipped with cyclotrons for producing the radionuclide.

The computer-reconstructed images of cross-sectional slices of the heart, shown in Figure 10, were obtained at the midventricular level. In the top panel is a transmission image. Radiation from a ring of positron-emitting material surrounding the patient is detected by an array of coincidence detectors rotated through 360 degrees. Solutions of the linear equations obtained from each positron permit computer reconstruction of an image reflecting transmitted radiation. The heart's location within the thorax is apparent in this cross-sectional image of the chest. In the bottom panel, an emission image was obtained after intravenous administration of

Figure 10. Positron-emission transaxial tomograms of the heart of a patient with acute myocardial infarction. (Courtesy of ES Weiss, MJ Phelps, EJ Hoffman, MM Ter-Pogossian, and BE Sobel.)

Transmission

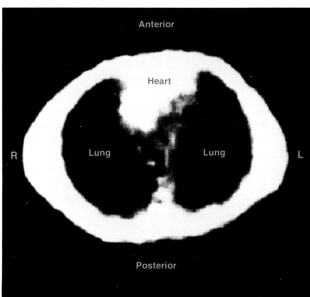

Emission $^{13}NH_3$

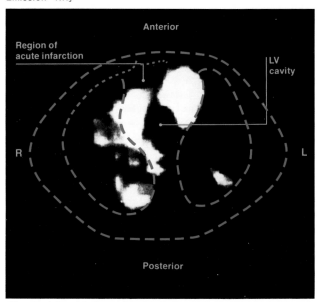

LV cavity: left ventricular cavity

^{13}NH$_3$, a positron-emitting radioisotope. Detection of the emitted radiation permits computer reconstruction of a transverse section at the midventricular level. The heart is clearly visible from radioactivity in the liver and spleen, which appears in regions overlapped by lung (outlined with a dashed line). A defect in the anterior portion of the ventricular wall corresponds to the site of myocardial infarction, detected by ECG. Such reconstructed images permit delineation of zones of altered metabolism indicative of ischemic injury *in vivo*.

In summary, current myocardial imaging techniques for the diagnosis of acute myocardial infarction appear promising; however, until the frequency of false-positive and false-negative diagnoses is determined, the practical utility of these techniques is uncertain. Additional studies will be required to determine whether a combination tracer technique (in which one tracer is administered to define a perfusion defect and another to define an area of increased radioisotope uptake) will enhance reliability and, therefore, utility.

SCINTIGRAPHIC EVALUATION OF LEFT VENTRICULAR FUNCTION

Radioactive tracers that remain in the circulating blood after injection, such as ^{99m}Tc-labeled serum albumin, can be used to define the left ventricular blood pool, which then provides the data from which end-systole and end-diastole can be measured.

The left ventricular ejection fraction can be calculated by scintigraphic techniques by dividing the end-diastolic volume minus the end-systolic volume by the end-diastolic volume.

The above method of calculating ejection fraction has been shown to correlate well with angiographic methods. Moreover, by defining the left ventricular blood volume throughout the cardiac cycle, regional abnormalities of wall motion can also be detected by scintigraphy (Figure 11). Assessment of segmental myocardial dysfunction may be aided by techniques that allow the data to be displayed in movie format. By this method, the left ventricle is visualized just as it is during contrast angiography. Several technological developments have allowed the use of this interesting technique during intense exercise. Hence, the means exist to measure global and segmental left ventricular function noninvasively at rest and during the stress of exercise. Preliminary data collected in our laboratory already suggest that, in contrast to normal individuals, ejection fraction diminishes during exercise in patients

Figure 11. Cardiac blood pool image obtained with technesium-labeled serum albumin injected intravenously. The labeled albumin defines the left ventricular cavity (right anterior oblique position) at end-diastole and end-systole. Figure 11(A) is a scintigram from a patient with a normal left ventricle. Figure 11(B) is a scintigram obtained from a patient with an area of akinesis involving the anterior apical left ventricular wall.

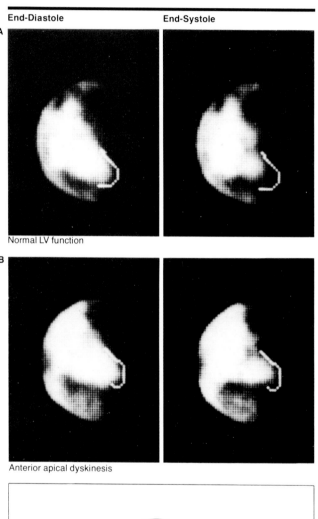

Normal LV function

Anterior apical dyskinesis

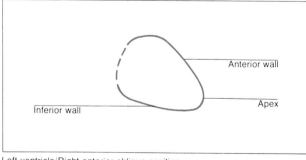

Left ventricle/Right anterior oblique position

with coronary artery disease. In addition, virtually all such patients develop abnormalities of left ventricular wall motion during exercise. These abnormalities appear even in those patients in whom left ventricle function is normal at rest.

The major advantages of isotopic scintigraphy over contrast angiography are (1) scintigraphic assessment of left ventricular contractile function requires intravenous injection of only the isotope; (2) it can be performed on an outpatient basis; and (3) it is free of the risks associated with left ventricular angiography. Thus, it safely and quickly provides information that can be used to assess long-term prognosis, advisability of operation, and changes in left ventricular function with time. In addition, cardiac blood-pool scintigraphic techniques have been useful in the screening of patients suspected of having left ventricular aneurysm. In such patients, a large localized blood pool with little or no change during the cardiac cycle is indicative of aneurysm. This finding aids in diagnosing coronary artery disease as well as in establishing the functional integrity of the left ventricle. Finally, easy assessment of segmental left ventricular function during exercise appears capable of providing a sensitive noninvasive screening technique for detection of CAD and may reveal whether a coronary lesion is functionally significant.

SECTION IV

Medical Treatment of Stable Angina Pectoris

Stephen E. Epstein, MD

Chief, Cardiology Branch
National Heart and Lung Institute
National Institutes of Health
Bethesda, Maryland 20014

Note: This chapter was written by Dr. Epstein in his private capacity. No official support or endorsement by the National Institutes of Health or the Department of Health, Education, and Welfare is intended or should be inferred.

Pathophysiologic Basis of Angina Pectoris

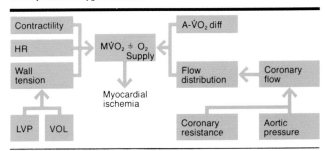

Figure 1. Determinants of myocardial oxygen supply and myocardial oxygen demand.

A-VO₂ diff: arteriovenous oxygen difference
HR: heart rate
LVP: left ventricular pressure

The physiologic basis for favorable results of treatment designed to reduce the discomfort of myocardial ischemia in coronary artery disease (CAD) patients can best be explained by considering the relative balance between delivery of, and demand for, myocardial oxygen. Because myocardial ischemia occurs when myocardial oxygen demand (MVO_2) exceeds the capacity of the diseased coronary vessels to deliver oxygen, therapeutic success depends on a favorable alteration of this balance. Either the coronary system's capacity for delivering blood to the ischemic regions of myocardium must be augmented, or myocardial oxygen demands must be reduced. Figure 1 depicts the major factors in this equation which, if unbalanced, will lead to myocardial ischemia. As can be seen, the major determinants of MVO_2 essentially depend on three factors: (1) the magnitude of systolic wall stress; (2) the frequency with which this stress is exerted; and (3) the contractile state of the heart.

FACTORS INCREASING AND REDUCING MVO_2

Wall stress depends on intraventricular pressure and, by the Laplace relationship, also upon ventricular volume; thus an increase in left ventricular pressure or volume will augment wall stress and, thereby, MVO_2. Likewise, a faster heart rate predisposes to ischemic pain because of greater oxygen needs. Finally, any intervention that increases myocardial contractility, in the absence of left ventricular failure, will lead to higher myocardial oxygen consumption. (When failure is present, however, a positive inotropic agent will also cause a diminution in left ventricular volume and end-diastolic pressure. These changes will affect the myocardial oxygen supply-and-demand ratio, by reducing MVO_2 and [as a consequence of reduction in left ventricular wall tension] by enhancing flow to ischemic myocardium.)

On the other side of the equation are those factors that alter myocardial blood flow, oxygen availability, and flow distribution. If coronary flow were decreased by a diminution in coronary perfusion pressure (as might occur with hemorrhage), myocardial ischemia might result. Similarly, any factors diminishing oxygen availability for a given rate of flow predispose to myocardial ischemia. This could result from anemia or from a shift in the oxyhemoglobin dissociation curve. Unfavorable shifts in oxyhemoglobin dissociation occur, for example, in response to carbon monoxide (an effect that may partially explain the deleterious effects of cigarette smoking on exercise performance). Favorable shifts in the oxyhemoglobin dissociation curve, making more oxygen available for any given PO₂ level, have been shown to occur in patients with cyanotic heart disease, myocardial ischemia, or congestive heart failure. Finally, nonhomogeneous distribution of flow across the myocardial wall occurs under physiologic conditions. This results in less endocardial than epicardial flow, and is exacerbated during acute episodes of myocardial ischemia. Endocardial flow decreases largely because myocardial wall tension is greater at the heart's endocardial surface than at the epicardial surface. This leads to greater compression of subendocardial coronary arterioles and collaterals, thereby increasing their resistance to flow. These factors help to explain the clinical and experimental observations that the endocardium is particularly vulnerable to the effects of ischemia.

An understanding of the factors responsible for maintaining the balance between myocardial oxygen supply and demand allows a more rational interpretation of the mechanisms responsible for precipitation of angina pectoris. For example, when exposed to low environmental temperatures, patients with CAD commonly experience angina pectoris while performing tasks that are well tolerated at more moderate temperatures. Studies show that exercise performed in the cold causes a greater increase in arterial pressure than an identical level of exercise performed at a more comfortable ambient temperature. Thus, the same intensity of exercise requires a higher level of MVO_2, a factor that undoubtedly contributes to the ease with which angina is precipitated in a cold environment. Marked rises in blood pressure are also observed even with localized exposure to cold, eg, after eating iced foods or immersing a hand in ice water. Apparently the autonomic responses to a cold environment can be triggered by exposure of only a small portion of the body surface to reduced temperature.

Hemodynamic changes leading to an increase in MVO_2, thereby predisposing to angina, also may be precipitated by anger, fear, and pain. Similar mechanisms contribute to the decreased exercise capacity that patients with angina pectoris experience after eating a meal. Several studies have shown that exercise performed after eating a 1,000 calorie meal is associated with a greater heart rate and mean arterial pressure than the same level of exercise performed under fasting conditions.

Nitroglycerin Therapy

One of the best known and most effective treatments for relieving pain caused by myocardial ischemia due to coronary artery disease is nitroglycerin administration. Nitroglycerin, given in amounts of 0.3 or 0.4 mg sublingually, consistently aborts the usual attack of angina pectoris. A fact often neglected is that *prophylactic* administration of nitroglycerin (ie, giving the medication a few minutes prior to an activity that usually provokes an anginal attack) is often effective in preventing the attack. For some patients, the prophylactic administration of nitroglycerin is particularly useful before entering into emotionally tense situations or before undergoing physical stresses, such as sexual intercourse, walking moderately long distances on a very cold day, playing golf, etc.

Since the introduction of nitroglycerin over a century ago, physicians have sought alternative forms of nitrate therapy that would extend the duration of antianginal effects. Nitrates with different molecular structures and different routes of administration have been used. Many of the so-called long-acting nitrates are in widespread use. The superiority of these agents over nitroglycerin in the treatment of angina pectoris remains unproven. For example, it has been claimed that sublingual isosorbide dinitrate (ISD) protects against the development of angina longer than does nitroglycerin.

One of the problems of comparing the relative efficacy of various drugs is the difficulty in choosing drug dosages. It is indeed possible to choose a dose of ISD that has a more prolonged antianginal effect than nitroglycerin. However, if this effect can be matched merely by increasing the dose of nitroglycerin, a conclusion that ISD has a more prolonged action would not be accurate. Obviously, the ideal way to assess the relative efficacy of two antianginal agents would be to perform dose-response curves until the *maximally tolerated* doses of each agent were reached and the resulting effects compared. However, this course is impractical and possibly dangerous. The technique we have employed is to choose drug doses on the basis of comparable physiologic responses; eg, nitroglycerin and ISD doses are selected that produce similar effects on heart rate and arterial pressure. When drug doses are chosen in this manner, and a standardized, reproducible exercise protocol is employed, sublingual nitroglycerin and sublingual ISD manifest virtually identical durations of action in their effects on the exercise capacity of patients with angina pectoris.

Nitroglycerin and structurally related nitrates also can be administered orally. One difficulty in achieving therapeutic effect by the oral route, however, is that nitrates are almost totally metabolized on their initial passage from the splanchnic circulation through the liver. It has been suggested that considerably larger doses of oral agents than have been traditionally used may allow enough intact drug to pass through the liver to achieve reasonable blood levels. Since it has been demonstrated *in vitro* that some nitroglycerin derivatives are metabolized more slowly than nitroglycerin itself, it has been suggested that these drugs, once in the systemic circulation, will have a prolonged action. However, it also has been shown that the more slowly metabolized nitrates are less potent vasodilators. Nevertheless, some data have been published demonstrating that oral administration of large doses of ISD (10 to 20 mg) have a longer duration of action than does sublingual nitroglycerin in preventing angina pectoris.

An alternative to changing the molecular structure of nitroglycerin, to achieve longer duration of action, might be to alter its mode of administration. The cutaneous application of nitroglycerin has been unequivocally demonstrated to be effective. Studies show that when nitroglycerin is applied to the skin in a lanolin base, the drug protects against the development of angina and enhances exercise capacity for over three hours. In clinical usage, the patient applies 0.25 inch or more of the ointment to a convenient area of the skin. The dose is gradually increased empirically until the patient first begins to feel a headache. The dose is then reduced just enough to avoid this undesirable side effect. Cutaneous application of nitroglycerin is particularly effective in patients experiencing nocturnal angina; application just prior to retiring usually prevents such occurrences. This long-acting preparation is also effective in preventing angina during such extended activities as golfing and hiking.

There are two potentially serious complications inherent in the administration of long-acting nitrate preparations: drug dependence and drug tolerance. Nitrate dependence, in which the body needs the drug to maintain physiologic homeostasis, is suggested by the experience of nitrate workers who develop headaches and other withdrawal symptoms during the weekend holiday when they are not exposed to nitrate. It has been suggested also that nitrate workers have an increased incidence of acute myocardial infarction. The postulated cause of such an event is the dependence of coronary arterioles on nitrates to maintain normal tone; when nitrate is absent, spasm ensues, with resultant diminution of myocardial flow.

Figure 2. Mechanisms of action of nitroglycerin.

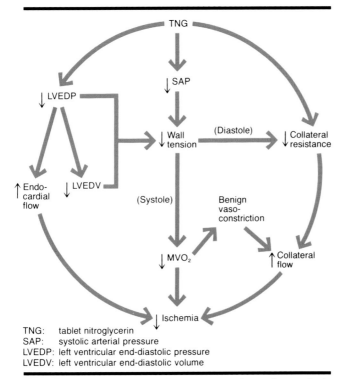

TNG: tablet nitroglycerin
SAP: systolic arterial pressure
LVEDP: left ventricular end-diastolic pressure
LVEDV: left ventricular end-diastolic volume

Anecdotal experience with patients on large doses of nitrates implies that nitrate tolerance, in which the body becomes resistant to the drug's pharmacologic actions, may develop. Neither drug dependence nor tolerance, however, has been documented in the clinical setting with patients given either sublingual or cutaneous nitroglycerin. Nonetheless, the physician must always be mindful of these potential complications as more widespread use is made of truly effective long-acting nitrate preparations.

MECHANISMS OF ACTION OF NITRATES

The beneficial effects of nitrates on myocardial ischemia are due to their complex influence on both myocardial oxygen requirements and myocardial oxygen delivery (Figure 2). They include the following:

Decreased MVO_2: Nitroglycerin reduces MVO_2 by diminishing left ventricular filling pressure and volume, thereby decreasing myocardial wall tension (and thus MVO_2) for any given level of systolic intraventricular pressure. Nitroglycerin also reduces myocardial wall tension by diminishing systolic arterial pressure.

Increased oxygen delivery: Nitroglycerin is able to reduce resistance to coronary collateral flow, to increase flow to the ischemic myocardium, and to produce a favorable redistribution of flow. Collateral flow and flow within the ischemic bed during diastole are probably increased in part by diminu-

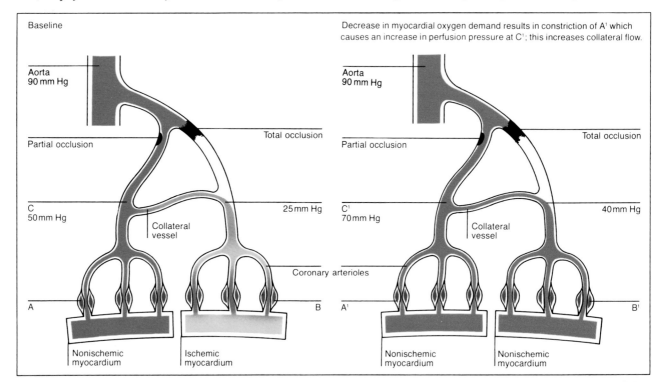

Figure 3. The figure depicts potential mechanisms that may lead to "benign" vasoconstriction. In this example, there is total occlusion of one coronary artery and partial occlusion of a second coronary artery, which is parallel to the first. The two coronary arteries are connected by a collateral channel. Muscles surrounding the coronary arterioles are depicted in brown. Control conditions are on the left and the response to a decrease in myocardial oxygen demands (MVO_2) is depicted on the right. The decrease in MVO_2 leads to constriction of the coronary arterioles supplying the nonischemic myocardium. This causes an increase in the perfusion pressure at the origin of the collateral vessel, leading to an increase in collateral flow.

Beta-Receptor Blockade

tion of ventricular diastolic volume and pressure. The associated decrease in wall tension would decrease the compressive forces on subendocardial arterioles and collateral channels, thereby enhancing flow to ischemic capillary beds. The decrease in MVO_2 of nonischemic myocardium produced by nitroglycerin probably results in metabolically mediated constriction of the arterioles supplying these beds. Since the arterioles supplying ischemic myocardium would remain dilated, perfusion pressure at the origin of collateral channels would increase, causing preferential shunting of blood from nonischemic to ischemic regions. This mechanism of action is depicted diagrammatically in Figure 3. It also appears likely that nitroglycerin causes direct dilation of coronary collateral channels. A direct enhancement of coronary collateral function has been demonstrated following intracoronary injection of nitroglycerin in patients with coronary artery disease who are undergoing coronary artery bypass surgery, as well as in experimental animals.

These favorable effects of nitroglycerin on MVO_2 and myocardial blood flow are somewhat offset by unfavorable hemodynamic alterations. Although the decrease in systolic pressure favorably alters MVO_2, the concomitant decrease in coronary perfusion pressure reduces myocardial blood flow and thus oxygen delivery. In addition, the reflex increase in heart rate, in response to reduction in arterial pressure, increases myocardial oxygen consumption. The decrease in diastolic filling time associated with the more-rapid heart rate also unfavorably influences myocardial blood flow.

Clearly, the net effect of nitroglycerin on myocardial ischemia is the result of its many influences on myocardial oxygen consumption and delivery. Given the clinical efficacy of nitroglycerin, it appears that the drug's deleterious effects are outweighed by its beneficial effects.

Stimulation of the cardiac sympathetic nerves and increased levels of circulating catecholamines result in an augmentation of heart rate and myocardial contractility. These changes predispose the patient to angina pectoris. Modulation of adrenergic drive to the heart by drugs capable of blocking beta-adrenergic receptors represents an important addition to the physician's armamentarium in the medical management of patients with angina pectoris. The efficacy of this approach has been demonstrated by many studies showing that propranolol reduces the frequency of anginal episodes, decreases the consumption of nitroglycerin tablets, and enhances exercise capacity.

It is important to emphasize that propranolol absorption varies considerably from patient to patient. Before conceding therapeutic failure, an adequate physiologic effect of the doses of propranolol employed should be demonstrated. Some patients require relatively large doses of propranolol to achieve the same reduction in exercise-induced tachycardia as is experienced by other patients receiving much smaller doses.

PATIENTS NEED EXPLANATIONS

To ensure that propranolol will be used in the safest and most effective way, it is important to explain carefully to the patient the expected benefits and the potentially dangerous side effects. The latter include shortness of breath, decreased exercise capacity, or more overt evidence of left ventricular failure. The patient should be instructed to stop taking the drug and call his physician if such side effects occur.

Once the patient understands this, propranolol is administered in relatively small doses: 10 mg four times a day. Thereafter, the dosage is increased by 40 mg per day every three to four days until a dose of 160 mg per day (in four divided doses) is attained. If this dosage results in appreciable symptomatic improvement and if the patient is able to perform most of his activities without the occurrence of angina, he continues to take 160 mg per day.

If, on the other hand, the patient still experiences frequent angina, dosage is gradually increased every few days in 40 mg increments to a daily dose of 240 mg; if improvement still is not evident, dosage can be increased to 320 mg or, very rarely, to 400 mg per day. If no improvement occurs at such high doses, blood levels of propranolol should be measured to determine whether the patient has an unusual problem of drug absorption. Most patients respond adequately to a total dose of 160 mg per day, but a small percentage of patients require either lower doses (80 mg per day) or somewhat higher doses (240 mg per day).

SIDE EFFECTS OF PROPRANOLOL

Although propranolol is effective in treating angina pectoris, it does have the potential for serious side effects. One is that removal of sympathetic inotropic support from a diseased myocardium can precipitate or exacerbate congestive heart failure. Thus, propranolol must be used with considerable caution in those patients who have significant myocardial dysfunction. Not only may such patients develop symptoms of congestive heart failure, but they also are the group least likely to experience relief of angina pectoris.

The great majority of patients with coronary artery disease who have no overt evidence of congestive failure do not develop failure when given propranolol. In the occasional patient who experiences congestive heart failure, however, it almost always can be controlled by concomitant administration of diuretics and, if necessary, digitalis. Propranolol should also be used with great caution in patients with asthma, since the loss of beta-receptor-induced bronchodilatation could lead to severe respiratory insufficiency.

An interesting and potentially serious side effect of abrupt discontinuance of propranolol has recently been noted. Some patients develop more-easily-precipitable angina, angina at rest, and even myocardial infarction and death upon abrupt withdrawal of propranolol. It also has been found that platelet aggregation is increased relative to the pretreatment state of the patient. This possibly may lead to acute increases in the severity of coronary occlusive disease. Alternatively, it is possible that such side effects are ascribable to an increased sensitivity of the beta receptor to a given level of sympathetic stimulation following prolonged inhibition of the receptor. Another potential cause for the observed complications following abrupt withdrawal is that patients raise their exercise limits to considerably higher levels when they are taking propranolol. If the drug is abruptly stopped after exercise has been increased, the effect is exposure of the patient to many more situations predisposing to the development of angina. Therefore, when propranolol is discontinued outside the hospital, it should be gradually decreased rather than abruptly withdrawn.

MECHANISMS OF ACTION OF BETA-RECEPTOR-BLOCKING DRUGS

Propranolol is thought to exert its effects in the following ways:

Decreased MVO_2: Reducing MVO_2 for any given level of activity increases the amount of exertion a patient can sustain before reaching the critical value of MVO_2 associated with the onset of ischemic chest pain. Beta-receptor blockade directly decreases the sympathetically mediated augmentation of heart rate and myocardial contractility that accompanies exercise. By diminishing myocardial contractility, propranolol also attenuates the exercise-induced increase in cardiac output, thereby modestly reducing the normal rise in blood pressure that occurs with exercise. Reductions in heart rate, contractility, and blood pressure all tend to lower MVO_2. However, beta-receptor blockade also increases ventricular volume, which tends to augment MVO_2. Clinical benefit from propranolol probably occurs because the oxygen-sparing effects of reduced heart rate, contractility, and blood pressure more than offset the additional oxygen costs imposed by an increase in ventricular volume.

Increased oxygen delivery: Theoretically, propranolol also acts to selectively augment blood flow to ischemic regions. By reducing MVO_2, propranolol would cause a metabolically mediated "benign vasoconstriction" in nonischemic regions, while producing little change in the areas that are ischemic. Reduction in MVO_2 benefits ischemic myocardium by helping to restore the balance between oxygen demands and limited oxygen supply. However, benign vasoconstriction of sufficient magnitude might also raise the pressure in nondiseased arterioles. If sufficient collateral channels arising proximal to the arterioles are available, this could result in a favorable redistribution of blood flow from nonischemic to ischemic regions (Figure 3).

COMBINED USE OF NITROGLYCERIN AND BETA-RECEPTOR BLOCKERS

Both the beta-receptor-blocking drugs and the nitrates have some circulatory effects that lower MVO_2. On the other hand, they have other circulatory effects that raise MVO_2, thus diminishing the beneficial effects. It is, therefore, of considerable therapeutic importance that beta-receptor-blocking drugs and nitrates have opposing circulatory influences that cancel the oxygen-wasting properties of the other (Table I). For example, the increase in ventricular volume produced by beta-receptor blockade, augmenting MVO_2, is opposed by the

Physical Conditioning

reduction in ventricular volume accompanying nitrate administration. Conversely, the sympathetically mediated rise in heart rate, reflexly induced by nitroglycerin, is attenuated by propranolol. Thus the combined administration of these two agents has a particularly favorable effect on exercise capacity.

DIGITALIS AND DIURETICS

Digitalis does not directly exert a favorable influence on angina in the absence of left ventricular failure. The added oxygen demand caused by the digitalis-induced increase in inotropic activity under these circumstances might actually worsen angina. Yet, in the presence of left ventricular failure, the decrease in ventricular volume accompanying digitalis treatment may cause a net decrease in MVO_2. Diuretics in the presence of failure would also reduce ventricular volume and thereby diminish MVO_2. The reduction in left ventricular volume and pressure would also decrease wall tension in diastole. This change might sufficiently reduce the forces compressing collateral vessels to increase flow to ischemic myocardia. Thus, digitalis and diuretics are important in the treatment of angina when the patient manifests signs or symptoms of left ventricular failure. In the absence of such symptoms, these drugs are ineffective and, in the case of digitalis, might actually prove deleterious.

Table I.
Complementary actions of nitroglycerin and propranolol on some of the determinants of myocardial oxygen supply and myocardial oxygen demand.

	Nitroglycerin	Propranolol
Ventricular volume	↓	↑
Diastolic wall tension	↓	↑
Systolic wall tension	↓	±
Heart rate	↑	↓

A patient's physical condition can significantly influence his circulatory response to exercise, thus altering his exercise capacity. Physical conditioning causes a lower heart rate and blood pressure response to a given level of exercise. As a result, the patient can perform more exercise before the critical or limiting MVO_2 is reached and angina precipitated. It has been postulated, although not proved, that exercise conditioning also enhances oxygen delivery to ischemic regions of the myocardium by stimulating growth of collateral vessels.

Regardless of the precise mechanisms involved, it is apparent that physical training results in a substantial increase in the exercise capacity of patients with angina pectoris due to coronary artery disease. The opposite of the conditioning process (a progressive reduction in activity level) leads to a diminution of exercise capacity. Thus, a timid patient (or physician) may initiate a vicious circle: excessive limitation of activity is prescribed because of angina, which leads to a reduction in exercise capacity that, in turn, ensures greater limitation of activity. This vicious circle can be broken only by restoring the patient's confidence that engaging in moderate activity (relative to his own maximum) is beneficial.

Before undertaking any conditioning program, the patient with CAD should exercise under the observation of a physician and with continuous ECG monitoring. If serious arrhythmias develop at the exercise loads that the patient would perform during the conditioning program, appropriate therapeutic measures should be initiated before the conditioning program begins.

What method is best for promoting good physical conditioning is somewhat controversial. A structured physical-activity class in a neighborhood gymnasium, administered by trained personnel and with resuscitation equipment available, is probably the optimal situation. However, most patients do not have access to such a facility. A regular program of jogging is an excellent physical-conditioning technique. It has some drawbacks, however: Excessively hot or cold weather may impose undue stress on some patients; in addition, minor and not-so-minor orthopedic complications are quite common. A possible alternative is for the patient to purchase a stationary bicycle, which would permit exercise to be performed at home in a comfortable environment. Bicycle exercise also eliminates the excessive stress that jogging imposes on the musculoskeletal system.

An additional benefit of a regular exercise program is the general feeling of well-being experienced by individuals in good physical condition. This sense of well-being often reduces background levels of anxiety, which in turn tends to reduce the frequency with which angina occurs. It should be emphasized, however, that imposition of an exercise program on an individual who has never exercised before, and who, in fact, dislikes exercise, may lead to adverse psychological and physical effects.

Finally, some patients do die suddenly during jogging or in an exercise class. Whether these events are causally related to the physical exertion or are merely coincidental is unknown. Nonetheless, the physician should be aware of the potential benefits as well as of the risks (however small) before prescribing an exercise program for an individual patient.

Summary:
An Approach to Treatment

The patient with angina pectoris should be evaluated for coexisting medical problems that might unfavorably influence his overall status. In particular, hypertension, hyperthyroidism, anemia, and tachyarrhythmias would all tend to augment myocardial oxygen consumption, thereby predisposing to the development of angina pectoris. If a patient is overweight, MVO_2 at any given level of exercise will be higher, contributing to impaired exercise capacity. If hyperlipidemia is present it should be treated.

Anxiety and tension should also be dealt with, not by routine administration of psychotropic agents but as part of a total approach to the patient's disease. This includes (1) a careful and complete explanation of why angina occurs and how it can be avoided; (2) a discussion of risk factors and the control of such factors as hypertension and hyperlipidemia; (3) a reassuring (but honest) opinion concerning the possibilities for the patient to lead a reasonably normal life for many years; (4) a description of the comprehensive medical approach planned for his problem and the chances of substantially reducing angina frequency; and, finally, (5) a discussion of the availability of operation, if this should become necessary.

Such an approach, in which the patient becomes a participant and not just a spectator in the planning of his therapy, almost invariably results in an improvement in his psychological (and therefore symptomatic) response to his disease.

Surgical Management of Atherosclerotic Vascular Disease

Atherosclerotic Occlusive Disease

Michael E. DeBakey, MD

President, Baylor College of Medicine
Chairman, Department of Surgery,
    Baylor College of Medicine
Director, National Heart and Blood Vessel
    Research and Demonstration Center
Houston, Texas

Charles H. McCollum III, MD

Assistant Professor of Surgery
Cora and Webb Mading Department of Surgery
Baylor College of Medicine
Houston, Texas

Atherosclerotic Occlusive Disease of the Coronary Arteries

Atherosclerotic occlusive disease of the coronary arteries produces symptoms of angina pectoris and acute myocardial infarction. The challenge of surgical treatment for coronary artery disease has intrigued surgeons for many years. Some of the surgical procedures that were pursued and have now been abandoned include induced myxedema, epicardial abrasion, internal mammary artery ligation, arterialization of the coronary sinus, and various neurosurgical procedures to produce cardiac denervation. Myocardial revascularization, using internal mammary artery implants into the ventricular myocardium, was introduced in the 1960s, but is rarely performed today.

In most instances, the atherosclerotic process is segmental in nature, with proximal occlusion or stenosis and a patent distal coronary artery. Coronary arteriography precisely determines the anatomical location of the disease. Once the occlusive process has been thus identified, revascularization may be individualized for each patient. Since 1963, when the first coronary artery bypass was performed in our institution using a reversed autogenous saphenous vein segment, this technique has become the standard surgical procedure for myocardial revascularization. It can be done simply and quickly, with good results, and immediately increases blood flow to the ischemic myocardium. In some patients, however, it may be necessary to perform an endarterectomy.

DIAGNOSIS

Atherosclerotic occlusive coronary artery disease is often first suspected during routine history-taking and physical examination. The patient may have a history of myocardial infarction or may have symptoms of angina pectoris. The resting electrocardiogram is often normal for patients with angina pectoris. Coronary arteriograms are indicated if a patient has intractable angina, angina after myocardial infarction, a positive exercise stress test, atypical chest pain, chest pain with valvular heart disease, or in a young patient who has sustained a myocardial infarction. Assessment of left ventricular function by combining left heart catheterization and ventriculography provides valuable information, including identification of areas of dyskinetic ventricular myocardium or ventricular aneurysms.

INDICATIONS FOR SURGERY

Surgery should be considered if there is coronary artery disease with a stenotic area greater than 70% in one or more

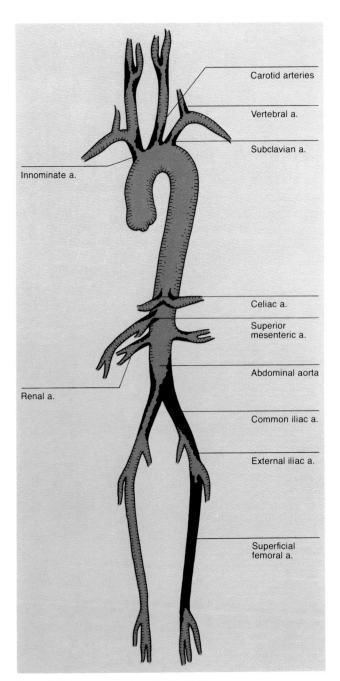

Figure 1. Patterns of occlusive vascular disease.

of the major arteries and a patent distal coronary vessel. Coronary artery bypass is also recommended for patients with intractable angina pectoris that cannot be controlled by medication. Patients with unstable angina (also known as crescendo or preinfarction angina) are also candidates for surgery.

Patients with high-grade stenosis of the left main coronary or proximal left anterior descending coronary artery represent "high-risk stenosis." Acute myocardial infarction and death are known to occur in this group, and surgical intervention is usually recommended. Ventricular septal defect, mitral insufficiency, and ventricular aneurysm may result from myocardial infarction. These may produce significant hemodynamic disturbances requiring surgical correction. Finally, some patients undergoing aortic valve replacement who have concomitant coronary artery disease should undergo coronary artery bypass. Patients with poor left ventricular function or congestive heart failure generally are not good candidates for coronary revascularization.

SURGERY

Patients undergoing cardiac surgery should be constantly monitored for changes in arterial blood pressure, electrocardiogram, central venous pressure (CVP), and temperature. Serial determinations of arterial blood gases, serum electrolytes, and hemoglobin are also carried out frequently. Endotracheal anesthesia is provided with nitrous oxide and oxygen, supplemented by thiopental sodium, muscle relaxants, and intravenous morphine.

The patient's saphenous vein is carefully removed through multiple incisions in the thigh. The vein is prepared by ligating its branches and removing any constrictive adventitia. The heart is exposed through a median sternotomy incision, the ascending aorta is cannulated, and venous catheters are inserted into the inferior and superior venae cavae through the right atrium. A left ventricular sump is inserted through the right superior pulmonary vein. A membrane oxygenator, primed with Ringer's lactate with 5% dextrose, is used for extracorporeal support. Cardiopulmonary bypass is instituted. Anoxic arrest, which provides a quiet heart without excessive bleeding, is achieved by cross-clamping the ascending aorta. The proper anastomotic site, distal to the occlusive lesion, is then located by examination of the coronary arteriograms and by palpating and inspecting the coronary arteries. Next, a longitudinal arteriotomy is performed, and the reverse saphenous vein autograft is sutured end-to-side to the coronary

artery, using a fine monofilament suture (Figure 2A, B). Endarterectomy of the right coronary artery is not often required.

After completion of the first distal coronary anastomosis, partial cardiopulmonary bypass is begun by releasing the aortic clamp and the caval tourniquets. A partially occluding vascular clamp is applied to the ascending aorta, and a longitudinal aortotomy is performed. The proximal anastomosis between the saphenous vein autograft and the aorta is carried out with an end-to-side anastomosis. With release of the partially occluding clamp, blood flow is routed through the coronary artery bypass to the distal coronary artery. The same technique can then be used for additional bypass grafts to

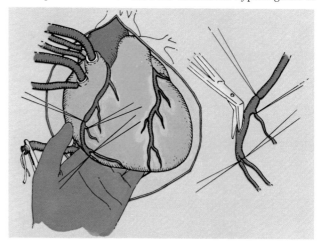

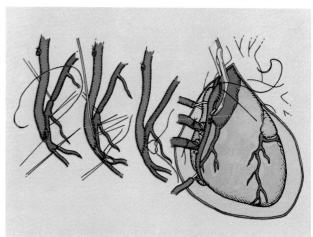

Figures 2A, 2B. Operative technique for right coronary artery bypass using autogenous saphenous vein and utilizing total cardiopulmonary bypass.

84

Figure 3. Coronary arteriograms, including seven-year follow-up of patient who underwent coronary artery bypass to left anterior descending coronary artery.

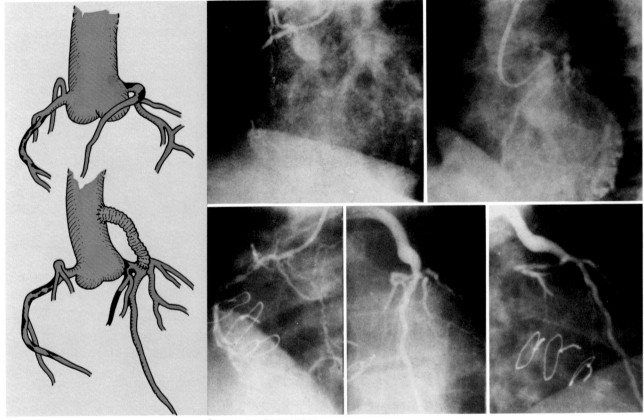

Seven years after operation

other segments of the coronary circulation. The grafts can be sutured proximally on the previously placed vein bypass graft or attached directly to the aorta.

Other necessary kinds of cardiac surgery are often performed at the time of coronary artery bypass. These include replacement of diseased cardiac valves and correction of any complications of preexisting coronary artery disease, such as mitral insufficiency from ruptured chordae or papillary muscle dysfunction, ventricular septal defects secondary to septal infarction, or aneurysms secondary to transmural infarction of the left ventricle.

RESULTS
Long-term patency of the saphenous vein bypass grafts de-

pends on the state of the distal coronary artery bed or "runoff" (Figure 3). Early patency rates are approximately 90%. Late occlusion of coronary artery bypass grafts may be caused by progression of the atherosclerotic process; it occurs in about 2% to 4% of cases annually. Operative mortality depends on the preoperative assessment of left ventricular function. In patients with normal left ventricular function, the mortality rate is about 2%, but impaired function increases the risk.

Many studies have reported beneficial effects from saphenous vein bypass, including symptomatic relief of chest pain or angina pectoris in many patients, as well as postoperative improvement in cardiac function in others. Evidence suggests that it decreases mortality from coronary artery disease and increases longevity.

Atherosclerotic Occlusive Disease of the Innominate, Carotid, Subclavian, and Vertebral Arteries

Atherosclerotic occlusive arterial disease may develop in the extracranial arterial circulation to the brain or upper extremities. However, surgical correction restoring a more normal cerebral blood flow is possible in more than one half of the patients with cerebral arterial insufficiency demonstrated by arteriography.

Extracranial occlusive arterial disease assumes a pattern of either proximal or distal occlusive disease. Proximal atherosclerotic occlusive plaques occur in the innominate, left common carotid, and left subclavian arteries of the aortic arch. Most patients with this form of the disease have multiple vessel involvement. The atheroma may be incomplete and well localized, or it may be complete, with a superimposed thrombus extending distally. However, since the atheromatous process rarely extends beyond the bifurcation of the common carotid artery, with proximal and distal vessels relatively normal, revascularization is possible in most cases.

In the distal form of the disease, the atheromas usually are located either in the internal carotid artery at the bifurcation of the common carotid or near the origin of the vertebral artery from the subclavian artery. Multiple lesions occur in most patients with vertebral artery occlusion and in approximately 70% of patients with internal carotid occlusion. Most patients in the earlier stages of the disease – manifested by transient ischemic attacks – show an incomplete and well-localized lesion, due to an atheroma near the origin of the internal carotid artery. This type of lesion can be treated surgically. In fact, surgery may at times prevent progression to an inoperable stage with the development of a permanent, serious neurological deficit.

Atherosclerotic occlusive disease of the brachiocephalic vessels occurs more often in men than women, with a ratio of 6:4. Approximately 90% of the time, it occurs in individuals during their fifties to seventies, although the age range is from 20 to 85 years. In younger patients, the occlusive process usually involves the vessels around the aortic arch. This form is more common in women and is frequently caused by arteritis rather than atherosclerosis.

SIGNS AND SYMPTOMS

There are many clinical manifestations of cerebral arterial insufficiency. They differ with the degree of occlusion and its location, the rate of progression of the occlusive process, and the extent of collateral circulation. There is abundant collateral communication around the circle of Willis and between branches of the external and internal carotid arteries. There is also communication among the branches of the thyrocervical trunk and those of the vertebral artery or the external carotid artery; these can provide additional pathways of collateral circulation.

Occlusion or stenosis of the internal carotid artery is often associated with ipsilateral monocular visual disturbances and contralateral motor and sensory deficits. The patient may be aware of a buzzing noise on the diseased side, corresponding to the bruit audible with a stethoscope. Occlusion or stenosis of the vertebral arteries may be associated with (1) bilateral visual disturbances; (2) vertigo; or (3) bilateral motor and sensory deficits, which occur first on one side and then on the other. Multiple lesions involving the carotid or vertebral system are common, causing some patients to have combinations of symptoms.

Symptoms may also be classified according to the characteristics of the attack. Patients with transient ischemic attacks have neurological disturbances which may last from a few seconds to several hours. The symptoms are short-lived and do not result in permanent neurological deficits. Such patients are ideal candidates for surgery since corrective surgery usually can be undertaken with excellent results.

Other patients may have neurological disturbances that persist or even progress over a period of hours or days. This pattern of symptoms is considered to be an evolving stroke. In general, unless these patients are seen very early in their clinical course, surgery should be postponed until they become more stabilized. Medical treatment may accelerate stabilization.

Other patients considered for surgical treatment are those with completed stroke, ie, a stable, persistent neurological deficit. Most of our patients with a completed stroke or a stroke in evolution have previously had symptoms of transient ischemic attacks and would have benefited from surgery. When the proper diagnosis is made early during the transient ischemic phase of the disease, the prognosis is better than after development of a progressing or completed stroke.

Other patients may have loud bruits or murmurs over the carotid artery, without symptoms of cerebral vascular insufficiency. Bruits usually indicate an obstructive atheromatous plaque. In general, if the patient has other significant cardiovascular disease that requires surgical intervention, we recommend arteriography and surgery. Otherwise, the bruits are not further treated in the asymptomatic patient.

Figure 4A-D. Surgical technique for carotid endarterectomy with patch angioplasty.

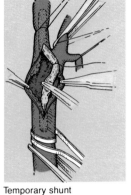
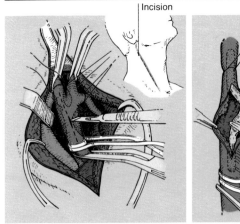

Incision

A.

Carotid artery incised

Temporary shunt inserted

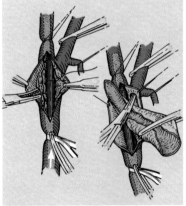
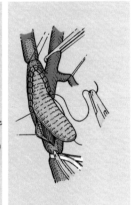

B.

Endarterectomy performed

Dacron patch sutured in place

The findings on physical examination depend entirely on the location and severity of the occlusive process. Some patients with transient ischemic attack may have no neurological findings; others have minimal-to-marked neurological deficits. Patients with proximal occlusive disease may have absent or diminished pulses in the neck and upper extremities. The brachial artery blood pressure may be reduced or unobtainable, and may be significantly different between the two arms. Bruits may be heard in the lower neck or supraclavicular fossa of patients with proximal innominate, common carotid, or subclavian occlusive disease, or in the anterior cervical triangle of patients with occlusive disease at the bifurcation of the carotid arteries. Occasionally, funduscopic examination reveals evidence of emboli, which may result from an ulcerative atherosclerotic plaque of the carotid artery.

A presumptive diagnosis of cerebrovascular insufficiency can be made based on the patient's symptoms and the results of physical examination; however, only angiography can establish an accurate diagnosis. We prefer the technique of bilateral percutaneous carotid and retrograde brachial vertebral arteriograms.

Arch aortography by the retrograde catheter technique is often performed on patients suspected of having proximal occlusive disease of the brachiocephalic vessels. Rarely, venous angioaortography may be indicated in patients with no accessible peripheral arteries in the arms or legs.

THERAPY

The goal of surgery is to restore normal circulation, thus relieving symptoms and preventing irreversible neurological damage. Endarterectomy and patch-graft angioplasty are appropriate for many of these lesions, particularly for stenosis of the internal carotid and vertebral arteries (Figures 4A-4D).

The following is an outline of a typical carotid endarterectomy: (1) the carotid bifurcation is approached via an oblique cervical incision along the anterior border of the sternocleidomastoid muscle; (2) temporary arterial clamps are placed on the exposed artery proximally and distally; (3) a longitudinal incision is made through the diseased segment under direct vision; (4) the atheromatous and diseased intima are carefully removed; and (5) the arterial incision is then closed with a patch, the edges of which are sutured circumferentially to the edges of the arterial wound. Our experience suggests that a temporary internal shunt reduces or prevents the

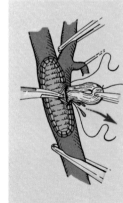
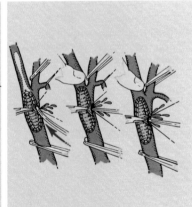

C.

Shunt withdrawn

Arteries flushed

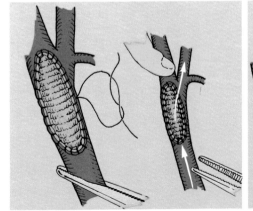
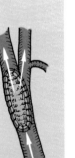

D.

Closure completed

effects of temporary cerebral ischemia in patients undergoing carotid artery surgery.

The more proximal occlusions of the great vessels originating from the aortic arch are preferentially treated by bypass graft technique. The ascending aorta is exposed through a second or third right anterior intercostal incision. A partially occluding clamp is applied to the ascending aorta, and one end of the graft is anastomosed end-to-side to the aorta. The patent distal arterial segments or segment is exposed through separate incisions in the neck and supraclavicular regions. The distal end of the graft is then drawn retrosternally through a tunnel made by blunt dissection and attached to a side of the patent distal vessel as an end-to-side anastomosis.

When multiple proximal occlusions are present, appropriate numbers of limbs are attached to the side of the original graft in the neck, while the other ends of the limbs are attached to the sides of other patent arterial segments. The knitted DeBakey Dacron velour tube grafts from 8 to 10 mm in diameter are ideal for use in grafts of the great vessels.

The bypass graft technique is also preferable for patients with localized occlusive disease of the common carotid or subclavian arteries. A carotid-subclavian bypass graft can be performed as an extrathoracic procedure, confining the operation to the neck or the supraclavicular regions, and avoiding a major intrathoracic operation. If a patient has occlusion of the left common carotid artery, one end of the tube graft can be attached to the side of a normal subclavian artery through a supraclavicular incision. The other end of the graft can then be attached to the patent carotid arterial segment distal to the occlusion through the same incision.

If the occlusion is localized to the proximal left subclavian artery, as in the subclavian steal syndrome, distal circulation can be provided by insertion of one end of the tubular graft to the side of a normal left common carotid artery in the neck, and the other end to the patent subclavian artery distal to the occlusion (Figure 5). This procedure corrects the reverse flow of blood from the basilar artery to the left vertebral and subclavian arteries.

The results of these surgical methods have been most gratifying. Since our first operation on August 7, 1953, we have treated over 5,000 patients. We have seen total operative mortality drop from approximately 6% to less than 2% and circulation improve in most patients who had suffered either occlusion or stenosis of the great vessels originating in the aortic arch or involving the origins of the internal carotid

Figure 5. Subclavian steal syndrome treated with left carotid-subclavian artery bypass graft.

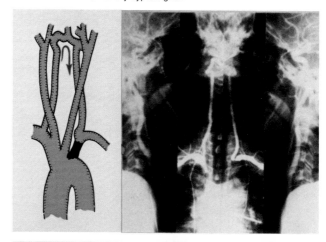

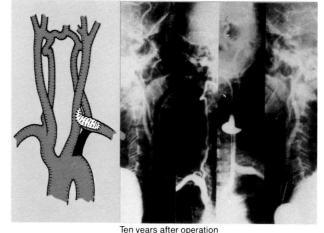

Ten years after operation

and vertebral arteries. Follow-up evaluation has shown relief of symptoms in approximately 95% of patients with transient cerebral ischemic attacks.

Notable in some patients with cerebrovascular insufficiency is the presence of associated cardiovascular atherosclerotic occlusive disease. In our experience, approximately 25% of patients operated on for cerebral arterial insufficiency have had associated disease of the abdominal aorta and of the iliac, femoral, popliteal, and renal arteries. Further, approximately 10% of patients with disease of the distal aorta have had extracranial occlusive vascular lesions as well. These

Atherosclerotic Occlusive Disease of the Renal Artery and Renal Vascular Hypertension

cases of multiple lesions demonstrate that atherosclerosis assumes multiple forms, even in the same patient. Each form, by proper treatment, may be corrected surgically. The occlusive disease affecting the cerebral arterial circulation is usually corrected first. Surgery is then performed in other occluded areas.

One form of hypertension that is surgically correctable results from atherosclerotic or fibromuscular hyperplastic narrowing of the renal artery. This possibility should be considered in all hypertensive patients, especially in those with an increase in, or a sudden onset of, the disease.

Atherosclerotic occlusive disease of the renal artery occurs more frequently in men; the male-to-female ratio is 9:1. Most affected patients are between 50 and 70 years old, although 23% of our patients have been younger than age 40. Fibromuscular hyperplasia of the renal arteries is most commonly seen in females under age 40. Patients with atherosclerotic occlusive disease of the renal artery may have other associated atherosclerotic occlusive disease in other areas. Many of our hypertensive patients with abdominal aortic aneurysms and occlusive disease of the abdominal aorta and iliac arteries show lesions of the renal arteries on aortogram. Both renal arteries may be affected; 40% of our hypertensive patients have bilateral disease.

Usually, the atherosclerosis involves only a short segment of the renal artery near its origin, with the distal segment being relatively normal. If the occlusive process is extensive or complete and the kidney has undergone secondary atrophy, nephrectomy is usually required. However, such kidneys can occasionally be preserved if collateral circulation from the capsular branches have maintained the patency of the distal arterial segments. When the occlusive process involves the branches of the renal artery, segmental or partial nephrectomy may be performed.

Occlusion of the accessory renal arteries occurs in approximately 10% of patients with renal vascular hypertension. These arteries are often small and, depending on the size and extent of the occlusion, surgical reconstruction may be difficult or impossible. In some patients, surgical revascularization or partial nephrectomy has been successful in relieving hypertension.

Many patients with renal artery stenosis have a systolic bruit in the upper abdomen or in the flank. Often there are no other signs to suggest the cause of hypertension. In evaluating the hypertensive patient, routine urinalysis is frequently negative, but may show albumen, red blood cells, or casts. (A more detailed discussion is presented in Section III.) The excretory urogram, particularly the hypertensive pyelogram, may show delayed excretion of contrast material and a decrease in the size of one kidney, suggesting renal vascular disease. Radioisotope studies, which provide a valuable noninvasive screening procedure, may suggest vascular abnormalities. Renal vein renin studies are becoming increasingly useful.

Aortography or retrograde selective renal arteriography is required for accurate diagnosis and for planning the surgical procedure. A criterion for surgery is the appearance of an anatomical obstruction of the renal artery in a hypertensive patient who has a significantly higher renal vein renin concentration on the affected side.

The aim of surgery is to ameliorate renal ischemia. Renal vascular reconstruction often can improve the blood supply and conserve renal tissue. Thin patients with well-localized disease are good candidates for endarterectomy and patch graft angioplasty. However, bypass is performed in most patients with extensive segmental lesions (Figure 6). The procedure is as follows: (1) the proximal end of the 6 mm DeBakey Dacron velour graft is attached to the abdominal aorta below the origin of the renal arteries; (2) the distal end of the graft is attached to the side of the renal artery distal to the area of occlusive disease; (3) the patent distal artery is preferably exposed by dissection outward from the aorta, although occasionally it may be necessary to reflect the colon medially. Bifurcation or separate grafts may be used for bilateral lesions. This may also be combined with aortoiliac grafting when indicated, in which case the proximal end of the renal artery graft is attached to the side of the aortic segment of the aorto-iliac bypass graft.

We have performed renal artery reconstructions in over 1,600 patients. Approximately 70% had atherosclerotic occlusive disease of the renal artery, whereas the rest had fibromuscular disease or renal artery aneurysms. Also, a small number of patients with uremia and renal artery occlusion have undergone surgery with resultant improvement in uremia.

The operative mortality in patients with renal artery stenosis has been reduced to approximately 4%. The major cause of death is myocardial infarction. After surgery, blood pressure has been significantly reduced in 86% of patients, and 57% have become normotensive. Most of the patients whose blood pressure was reduced, but who did not become normotensive, have had residual systolic, rather than diastolic, hypertension. Follow-up arteriograms were obtained in over half of the patients with renal vascular hypertension. Occlusion of the renal artery bypass occurred in 5% of the reconstructed cases, requiring secondary revascularization or nephrectomy.

Figure 6. Bilateral renal artery bypass using Dacron tube grafts, performed in 1964 on patient with renovascular hypertension who has remained normotensive since surgery.

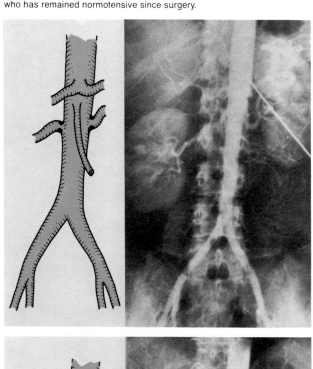

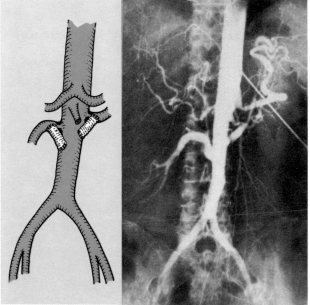

Ten years after operation

90

Atherosclerotic Occlusive Disease of the Splanchnic Arteries

CELIAC, SUPERIOR MESENTERIC, AND INFERIOR MESENTERIC ARTERIES

Acute arterial mesenteric occlusion is a severe disease which is fatal if not properly treated. Fortunately, about half of the patients with preexisting atherosclerotic occlusive disease of the splanchnic vessels have warning symptoms of pain, called "abdominal angina."

The symptom complex of abdominal angina is fairly characteristic. The patient has crampy postprandial pain located in the epigastrium. The pain may last for one to three hours, often radiating to the back. Other symptoms include significant weight loss, anorexia, nausea, vomiting, bloating, diarrhea, or constipation. Physical examination may also reveal an abdominal systolic bruit. Our experience has shown that many patients with these symptoms have occlusive or aneurysmal disease in other areas of the vascular tree as well. If mesenteric insufficiency is properly diagnosed and surgical revascularization performed, the symptoms may be relieved and the disaster of mesenteric arterial thrombosis with infarction of the bowel prevented.

Many patients have concomitant angina pectoris, intermittent claudication, or symptoms of cerebrovascular insufficiency. The splanchnic atheroma is usually located in the first 2 to 3 cm of the involved vessel, with a patent distal segment which is amenable to reconstructive vascular surgery. Occlusive disease is common in at least two of the three vessels (celiac, superior mesenteric, and inferior mesenteric arteries).

DIAGNOSIS

A diagnosis of mesenteric insufficiency or abdominal angina must obviously exclude other gastrointestinal disorders. Routine roentgenograms of the gastrointestinal tract are often negative, although puddling of the barium may be seen in the intestine. Occult blood is frequently present in the stool. Some patients have findings of malabsorption syndrome with a decreased excretion of D-xylose and increased loss of fecal fat. A standard aortogram should be done if other vascular abnormalities are suspected. In the posteroanterior projection, the aortogram may show evidence of an enlarged inferior mesenteric artery providing collateral circulation to the mesenteric vascular bed. To adequately visualize the celiac and superior mesenteric arteries, an aortogram or selective arteriograms must be obtained in the lateral projection.

The operation for mesenteric insufficiency is designed to revascularize the splanchnic arterial bed to restore normal circulation, thus eliminating the symptoms of abdominal angina and avoiding acute mesenteric occlusion. Endarterectomy can occasionally be performed, but the difficulty encountered in exposing the origin of the superior mesenteric and celiac arteries makes this method less desirable. The bypass graft technique has provided quite satisfactory results (Figure 7). A long midline abdominal incision is used, and the infrarenal abdominal aorta is exposed. A partial occluding clamp is applied and the proximal end of the graft is attached end-to-side to the aorta. It can then be tunneled behind the transverse mesocolon and stomach and anastomosed end-to-side to the splenic or hepatic artery. The disease usually spares the trifurcation of the celiac artery and good revascularization of the entire celiac bed is thus possible. A tube graft can be sutured end-to-side from the initial graft, then tunneled through the small bowel mesentery and sutured end-to-side to the superior mesenteric artery distal to the origin of the middle colic artery. DeBakey Dacron velour grafts of 6 to 8 mm diameter have been most satisfactory. Autogenous saphenous veins have been used occasionally.

Approximately one half of our patients have undergone concomitant vascular surgical procedures, including resection of an abdominal aortic aneurysm, or bypass grafting for aortoiliac occlusive disease or renal artery stenosis. Occasionally, the proximal end of the mesenteric artery bypass originated from an abdominal aortic graft. Results of mesenteric artery revascularization have been excellent. The majority of our patients have had their symptoms relieved and their lives greatly prolonged.

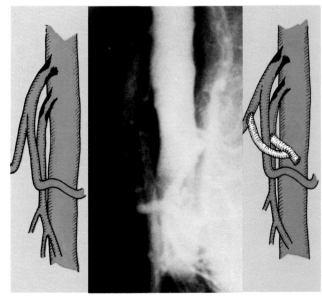

Figure 7. A patient with classical symptoms of abdominal angina treated successfully using a bypass graft from the abdominal aorta to the hepatic and superior mesenteric arteries.

Atherosclerotic Occlusive Disease of the Abdominal Aorta and the Iliac Arteries

The Leriche syndrome is the familiar term for atherosclerotic occlusive disease of the aorta and iliac arteries. Atheromatous changes are usually found in the terminal abdominal aorta and common iliac arteries and may spread distally to encroach on the bifurcation of the iliac artery. The atheromatous process causes reduction in the size of the vessel lumen and a decrease in the arterial blood flow. Ultimately, as the flow is retarded, thrombosis with complete obstruction of the aorta can occur. With gradual occlusion of the aortoiliac segment, collateral circulation may develop around the area of obstruction.

If occlusion of both iliac arteries occurs, superimposed thrombus causes complete occlusion of the distal aorta and expands proximally toward the renal arteries. This form of atherosclerotic occlusive disease in the aortoiliac segment is seen predominantly in men, with a male-to-female ratio of 10:1. Ninety percent of our patients are between 50 and 70 years old; the youngest was 23 years old and the eldest, 90.

The clinical manifestations of the disease depend upon the site, extent, and duration of the occlusive process. If the process develops slowly, extensive collateral circulation has time to develop. These collateral channels may minimize symptoms, but will not eliminate them. When the occlusive process occurs acutely, without time for collateral circulation to develop, distal circulation may be impaired quite suddenly, with severe symptoms of ischemia to the lower extremity. Fortunately, most patients develop the occlusion gradually.

The first clinical manifestation is usually intermittent claudication in the buttocks, thighs, or calves, which produces pain during exercise that is relieved by rest. Sexual impotence may develop in affected males. As the occlusion becomes more severe, the patient may develop nocturnal pain as well as pain at rest. The muscle mass of the lower extremities and the subcutaneous tissue undergo atrophy, hair is lost, and toenails show evidence of hypertrophy. Ultimately, pregangrenous or gangrenous changes may occur on the skin of the feet. Diagnosis can be suggested by noting the diminution or absence of pulses over the femoral, popliteal, and pedal arteries. Also, systolic bruits may be heard over the lower abdominal aorta and in the inguinal areas. Thirty percent of patients with proximal aortoiliac disease also have distal occlusive disease in the superficial femoral, popliteal, or tibial vessels. A large number have renal artery occlusive disease sufficient to produce associated hypertension.

These symptoms justify a presumptive diagnosis of Leriche syndrome. However, aortograms are needed to establish a positive diagnosis and to determine the extent of disease. Appropriate surgery then can be selected. We prefer to perform our aortograms under general anesthesia, using the percutaneous translumbar route with the patient in the prone position (Figure 8). The translumbar aortogram needle is introduced below the left twelfth rib, just lateral to the paraspinous muscles, and is inserted into the aorta at the level of the twelfth thoracic or first lumbar vertebra; 35 ml of iothalamate meglumine is then injected. A 36-inch cassette is used to allow visualization of the abdominal aorta and the common and superficial femoral arteries. For better visualization of the distal arterial circulation in the leg, the patient is then placed in the supine position. Bilateral percutaneous femoral angiography is performed using 35 ml of 50% sodium diatrizoate injected in each leg. This method of angiography has few complications and provides good visualization of the superficial femoral, popliteal, and tibial vessels.

Fortunately, because of the segmental nature of proximal atherosclerotic occlusive disease, distal circulation can be improved or restored in virtually all patients. A vessel distal to the aortoiliac occlusion is nearly always available: the external iliac, common femoral, profunda femoris, or popliteal artery. Furthermore, advanced age, hypertension, compensated heart disease, and diabetes are not definite contraindications to surgery. In our large group of patients undergoing surgical correction for aortoiliac occlusive disease, almost one half have been hypertensive, one third have had heart disease, and one tenth have been diabetic.

The method of arterial reconstruction elected at the time of operation is based on an evaluation of preoperative arteriograms and the operative findings (Figure 9). If the atherosclerotic occlusive process is localized to the terminal abdominal aorta and proximal common iliac arteries, and is confined to the intima, then thromboendarterectomy may be carried out. This procedure is performed through separate transverse incisions in the aorta and the common iliac arteries. The proper cleavage plane between the diseased intima and the more normal outer layers is entered, and the occlusive atheroma is removed, using blunt dissection. In larger vessels, vascular continuity can be restored by simple closure of the arterial incision. Another surgical technique is to perform an aortotomy across the localized atherosclerotic plaque and to close the incisions by inserting a patch graft angioplasty. The edges of the Dacron patch are sutured circumferentially

Figure 8. Technique for translumbar aortogram
performed under general anesthesia in prone position.

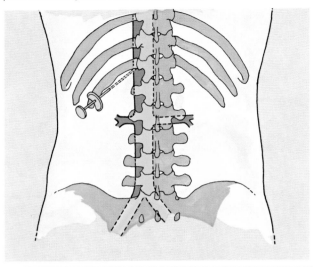

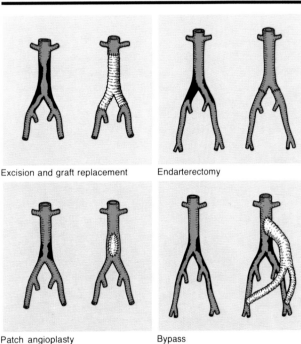

Excision and graft replacement   Endarterectomy

Patch angioplasty   Bypass

Figure 9. Techniques for surgical management of atherosclerotic occlusive
disease of aortoiliac segment.

to the edges of the arterial wound by simple over-and-over
sutures.

A third method of arterial reconstruction, excision, and graft
replacement is used in patients who have aortoiliac occlusive
disease associated with aneurysms of the abdominal aorta.
With this method, the diseased segment is excised and replaced with a suitable DeBakey Dacron bifurcation graft. The
proximal anastomosis is usually performed several centi-
meters below the renal artery by an end-to-end anastomosis.
The distal anastomosis is carried out between the limbs of
the bifurcation graft and the appropriate distal artery, either
the common or the external iliac artery. If the disease process

is more extensive, it may be necessary to perform an anastomosis distal to the inguinal ligament, to either the common
femoral or profunda femoris artery.

In most patients with Leriche syndrome, a fourth method,
the bypass graft technique (Figure 10), is preferred. A knitted
DeBakey Dacron graft is used and the proximal end of the graft
is attached to the uninvolved aorta above the obstructive
disease and below the renal arteries. An appropriate retroperitoneal tunnel is made, through which the graft is passed distally. The limbs of the bifurcation graft can then be sutured by
an end-to-side anastomosis, distally to a patent segment of the
external iliac, common femoral, or profunda femoris artery.
Occasionally, it is necessary to extend the distal anastomosis
to the popliteal artery. If the patient has associated occlusive disease of the superficial femoral artery, a simultaneous
femoral-popliteal bypass graft can be performed. Rarely, patients have unilateral iliac occlusive disease that requires
only a straight tube graft. Most patients have atheromatous involvement of both common and external iliac arteries, and require a bifurcation graft.

For some patients it is desirable to avoid an intra-abdominal
procedure, specifically those patients in poor medical condition or those who may have intra-abdominal sepsis or infection of a previously placed vascular graft. Revascularization
of the lower extremity can be achieved by using a crossover
femoral-to-femoral artery bypass graft if the patient has unilateral iliac occlusive disease.

In some cases of bilateral iliac occlusive disease, a bypass
graft from the axillary artery to the common femoral artery
is performed via a subcutaneous tunnel from the axilla to the
groin. Once this bypass is performed, it may then be possible to use a cross-over, femoral-to-femoral artery graft to the
contralateral femoral artery. If superficial femoral artery
disease is present, the distal limb of the axillary graft may
be anastomosed to the popliteal artery above the knee.

Our operations for aortoiliac occlusive disease have generally been very successful, with an overall operative mortality less than 2%. Successful pulse restoration, avoidance of
amputation, and relief of symptoms have been obtained in
98% of the survivors. Follow-up evaluations on patients,
extending up to two decades in some instances, have indicated that the early results have been maintained. However,
while complications are rare, graft thrombosis, hemorrhage,
and graft infection do occur occasionally and require secondary surgical procedures.

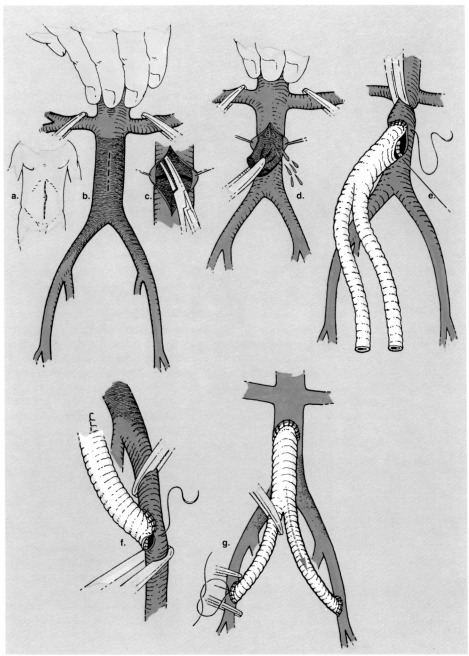

Figure 10. Steps in operation technique for correction of extensive aortoiliac occlusive disease.

a. Incision
b. Aorta isolated
c. Aortotomy made
d. Thrombectomy performed
e. Dacron bifurcation graft anastomosed end-to-side to aorta
f. Left limb of graft anastomosed to left external iliac artery
g. Right limb of graft anastomosed to right iliac artery

Atherosclerotic Occlusive Disease of the Superficial Femoral, Popliteal, and Tibial Arteries

Atheromatous involvement of the superficial femoral, popliteal, or tibial vessels may be associated with either complete or partial occlusion. The occlusion is most commonly located in the distal superficial femoral artery near the adductor canal, with uninvolved proximal and distal segments of arteries. In some cases, the atherosclerotic process may be more widespread, extending from the common femoral to the popliteal artery. Further distal extension of the atheromatous process may involve the popliteal artery or its branches.

Most patients with atherosclerosis of the superficial femoral or popliteal artery are amenable to surgical revascularization. These patients usually have intermittent claudication of the calf, rather than of the thigh or buttocks, as occurs in aortoiliac occlusive disease. More severe ischemic manifestations are present because the obstructive process is more distal in the arterial tree, which allows for a less-satisfactory development of collateral circulation. Many patients with more extensive tibial disease are not suitable for the standard femoral-popliteal bypass graft. However, application of the bypass graft to the tibial or peroneal arteries has proved successful if there is a patent vessel. Patients with the tibial pattern of distal occlusive disease often have pain at rest at night or trophic cutaneous changes. The popliteal and pedal pulses are usually diminished or absent.

Although the diagnosis usually can be made on the basis of characteristic clinical manifestations, the extent of the obliterative process does not always correlate well with the degree of ischemia. Some patients with extensive atherosclerotic occlusive disease not amenable to surgery may have only intermittent claudication. Others, with more localized, discrete lesions that are easily corrected surgically, may show signs of severe ischemia, including gangrene. Thus, arteriography is essential for all patients, to determine the exact location and extent of the disease. Aortography should be performed to exclude any unsuspected proximal aortoiliac occlusive disease that may retard blood flow through the grafts inserted in the femoral-popliteal segment during surgery. Also, an unsuspected aneurysm of the abdominal aorta may occasionally be discovered. Percutaneous femoral arteriography is then performed as previously described. This indicates the location and extent of the occlusive disease and, most importantly, the "distal runoff." A good runoff demonstrates the patency of the distal arterial tree favorable to supporting a bypass graft. Femoral arteriograms reveal patent distal segments favorable for operation in approximately 90% of patients with symptoms of intermittent claudication. However, in patients with more severe symptoms (pain at rest, gangrene, and consequently more extensive atherosclerotic occlusive disease), only about 50% have distal segments favorable for bypass surgery. Aside from these anatomical findings, the major contraindication is an untreatable disease that limits activity or life expectancy. If severe ischemia has already produced obvious gangrenous changes, early amputation may be indicated.

The type of surgery required depends upon the arteriographic findings. Short, localized segments of occlusive disease may be amenable to endarterectomy and patch graft angioplasty. The involved artery is exposed, so that temporary occluding clamps can be applied across a normal artery above and below the obstruction. A longitudinal incision is made through the region of obstruction under direct visualization; the diseased intima is then removed from the main central channel and from the orifices of the arterial branches arising from this segment. The arterial incision is closed with insertion of a patch graft, using simple continuous sutures.

When there is extensive involvement of the femoral-popliteal arterial segment, the bypass technique is preferred. This technique avoids extensive dissection and damage to existing collaterals and provides a simpler operative procedure. Through a small groin incision, the common femoral artery is exposed. The proximal end of a 6 or 8 mm DeBakey Dacron velour graft is sutured to the common femoral artery with an end-to-side anastomosis using simple over-and-over sutures (Figure 11). The graft is then tunneled, in the subfascial plane, into the popliteal fossa made by a second incision employed to expose the popliteal artery above the knee. An end-to-side anastomosis between the distal end of the graft and the popliteal artery is then carried out, restoring blood flow. Operative arteriograms are routinely employed to identify immediately any emboli that may lie in the distal vessels, or any constriction at the site of the distal anastomosis. Such problems can be corrected at the time of surgery.

If the atheromatous process extends more distally, and if the distal anastomosis is required below the knee, the reverse autogenous saphenous vein graft is preferred and provides satisfactory results. If the popliteal trifurcation is involved, the distal tibial artery bypass may be employed. Using an autogenous saphenous vein, the distal anastomosis is then carried out to the distal tibial or peroneal arteries.

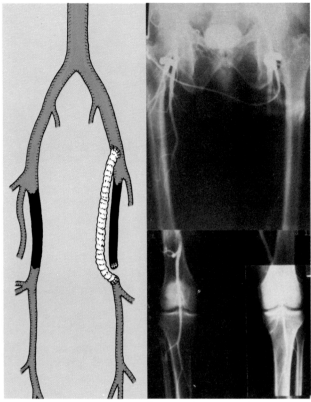

Ten years after operation

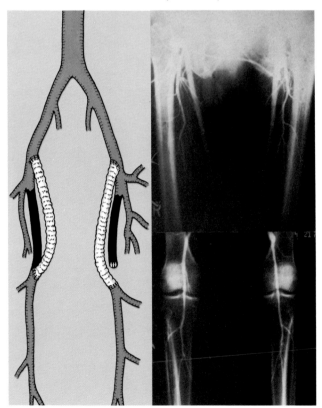

Four years after operation

Figure 11. Patient has intermittent claudication of both calves. Top: Femoral-popliteal bypass graft performed in 1962. Bottom: Femoral-popliteal bypass performed in 1968. Both grafts patent and functioning 10 and 4 years after insertion, respectively.

One may expect a 60% patency rate of these distal tibial artery grafts. If the grafts remain open for three to six months in patients with severe pain at rest or with gangrenous changes, these open wounds usually heal and collateral circulation is improved, providing continued relief of symptoms and salvage of the extremity. This is true even if graft closure occurs at a later date.

Some patients have extensive, diffuse obstructive disease of the popliteal and tibial arteries that is not suitable for reconstructive surgery. These patients are considered for lumbar sympathectomy, a procedure that can be combined with aortic, iliac, or femoral reconstructive surgery. This procedure may also allow the healing of gangrenous changes or ischemic ulcers.

Relief of symptoms and restoration of a more normal distal circulation can be obtained in a high proportion of patients using the femoral-popliteal bypass technique. Surgical reconstruction has been feasible in approximately 90% of our patients with superficial femoral artery occlusive disease, using the 6 and 8 mm DeBakey Dacron velour grafts from the common femoral artery to the popliteal artery above the knee. Patency rates similar to those obtained with vein bypass grafts at the same sites have been obtained. Our patency rates have been 83%, 73%, and 69% after one, three, and five years, respectively. We therefore use the DeBakey Dacron velour graft for bypasses above the knee, and reserve the saphenous vein for popliteal and tibial artery bypasses below the knee. We have found that the incidence of recurrent occlusion is higher in the femoral-popliteal area than in the more proximal aortoiliac occlusive disease. This complication is due to (1) progression of proximal aortoiliac lesions, (2) progression of more distal disease, and (3) technical factors related both to the underlying disease and to the operation performed. Even when recurrent occlusion occurs, a significant number of patients do have a patent distal segment which permits reoperation and restoration of improved circulation. Despite the higher incidence of recurrent occlusion in this area, in many cases surgical reconstruction is the only method that will relieve symptoms and reverse ischemic damage that would otherwise require amputation. For this reason, an aggressive approach to these problems seems justified.

ACKNOWLEDGMENTS

The following figures have been reproduced by permission of the authors and publishers.

Figure 1. DeBakey ME, Beall AC Jr: Surgical treatment of diseases of the aorta and major arteries, in Hurst WJ, Logue RB (eds): *The Heart,* ed 2, 1970, p 1534. Courtesy of McGraw-Hill Book Co Inc, New York, NY.

Figures 2A and 2B. DeBakey ME, McCollum CH III: Coronary artery bypass procedures. *Comp Ther* 1:16-17, 1975. Courtesy Book Assoc Int'l, Harvard, MA.

Figure 3. Garrett HE, Dennis EW, DeBakey ME: Aortocoronary bypass with saphenous vein graft seven-year follow-up. *JAMA* 223:793, 1973. Copyright 1973, American Medical Association.

Figure 10. Garrett HE, Crawford ES, Howell JF, et al: Surgical considerations in the treatment of aortoiliac occlusive disease. *Surg Clin North Am* 46:960, 1966. Courtesy WB Saunders Co, Philadelphia, PA.

Surgical Management of Atherosclerotic Vascular Disease

Atherosclerotic Aneurysmal Disease

Michael E. DeBakey, MD

President, Baylor College of Medicine
Chairman, Department of Surgery,
    Baylor College of Medicine
Director, National Heart and Blood Vessel
    Research and Demonstration Center
Houston, Texas

Charles H. McCollum III, MD

Assistant Professor of Surgery
Cora and Webb Mading Department of Surgery
Baylor College of Medicine
Houston, Texas

98

Classification of Aneurysms

Untreated aneurysms of the aorta tend to enlarge and ultimately produce serious or even lethal complications from rupture and exsanguination, or from compression of surrounding tissues. During the past few decades, successful surgical techniques have been developed for managing aneurysmal disease.

Aneurysms may be classified according to location, morphology and etiology. Aneurysms tend to assume specific patterns, depending on their location (Figure 1). The most common form involves the abdominal aorta, arising just distal to the renal arteries and extending to the bifurcation of the common iliac arteries. Second in frequency are aneurysms of the descending thoracic aorta, arising just distal to the left subclavian artery. Other common sites of involvement are the ascending aorta, transverse arch and thoracoabdominal segment, in that order.

Morphologically, aneurysms may be classified into three types: *fusiform*, encompassing the entire circumference of the aorta and assuming a spindle shape; *sacciform*, or narrow-necked, pouch-like protrusions from the aortic wall; and *dissecting*, distinguished by an intramural separation, usually within the medial layer.

Dissecting aneurysms may be further classified into three subtypes: (1) those that begin in the ascending aorta and extend distally, often as far as the abdominal aorta and iliac arteries; (2) those that also originate in the ascending aorta, but are limited to the ascending aorta proximal to the innominate artery; and (3) those that originate distal to the subclavian artery and may be localized to the descending thoracic aorta, or may extend below the diaphragm.

Aneurysms may be caused by atherosclerosis, infection or trauma, or related to congenital abnormalities, or by previous vascular surgery. Atherosclerosis is the most prevalent single cause. Appropriate antibiotic therapy has reduced significantly the incidence of aneurysms caused by syphilitic infections. Aneurysms of the descending thoracic aorta are seen more and more as a result of blunt trauma to the chest. (The blow usually produces a tear in the aortic wall near the upper descending thoracic aorta which, if unrecognized initially, may develop into an aneurysm.)

Rare congenital aneurysms are related to other inherited anomalies, such as coarctation of the aorta or patent ductus arteriosus. An occasional false aneurysm may develop at the site of a previous aortic anastomosis with a prosthetic graft. Cystic medial necrosis, sometimes associated with Marfan's syndrome, may be a cause of aneurysmal disease of the dissecting type occurring in the thoracic aorta.

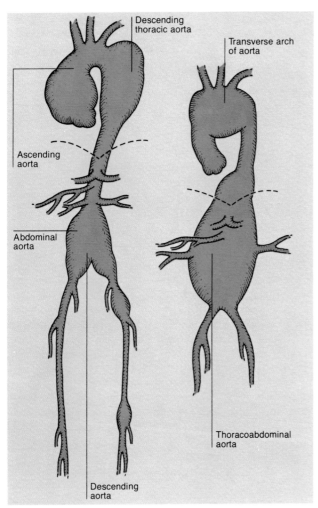

Figure 1. Patterns of aneurysmal vascular disease.

Aneurysms of the Thoracic Aorta

Clinical manifestations of aneurysms of the thoracic aorta are related to intramural aortic dissection, rupture, or expansion. They may also be related to distortion, compression, and erosion of surrounding structures. The blood-filled sacs sometimes enlarge slowly and progressively without producing symptoms, and are discovered only by routine chest x-rays. They may occur at any age. In younger patients they are usually present in the ascending aorta, because of the higher incidence of cystic medial necrosis. However, in the descending thoracic aorta, most of the aneurysms are atherosclerotic in origin and occur in patients who are 60 to 70 years old. Men are affected nine times more often than women. Atherosclerotic aneurysms or occlusive disease may be present as coexisting disease in different locations of the arterial tree. Careful evaluation of the patient is suggested.

Pain is certainly the most common symptom of an aneurysm. It may be gradual as the aneurysm enlarges, or may become more acute, as in the dissecting aneurysm or in one that is expanding or leaking. The pain may be in either the substernal or in the intrascapular area. It often radiates to the neck, shoulders, or abdomen. Increasing intensity and amount of pain is an ominous sign which may indicate a rapid enlargement or impending rupture.

Aneurysms of the ascending aorta may also have associated aortic valvular insufficiency. Respiratory difficulty may result from compression or distortion of the trachea. Hoarseness, caused by infringement of an expanding aneurysm on the left recurrent laryngeal nerve, with paralysis of the vocal cord, is a common symptom. Esophageal compression may also lead to dysphasia. Neurological symptoms from spinal cord ischemia may occur, especially in patients with a dissecting thoracic aneurysm. Rupture of an aneurysm of the thoracic aorta usually results in sudden death from hypovolemic shock. Symptoms of a ruptured aneurysm vary, depending upon the site and extent of the rupture. Hemoptysis and hematemesis may occur with rupture and communication between the aneurysm and the tracheobronchial tree or the gastrointestinal tract. Cardiac tamponade may be seen with rupture or leaking into the pericardium. However, a few patients with aneurysms may have only one of these symptoms.

Thoracic aneurysms are usually not detected on physical examination. Occasionally, however, it may be possible to observe or palpate a pulsation above the suprasternal notch, or at other sites in the chest because of erosion through the thoracic cage. Aortic valvular insufficiency may occur from progressive annular dilatation associated with aneurysms of the ascending aorta or from acute prolapse of the aortic valve associated with dissecting aneurysm. The peripheral pulses are usually normal, but may be reduced or absent with dissecting aneurysms. Tracheal deviation may be identified in patients with thoracic aneurysms. In most cases, plain posteroanterior and lateral roentgenograms of the chest will show enlargement of the involved aortic segment. Calcification in the aneurysmal wall may also be visualized roentgenographically. Widening of the mediastinum or hemothorax may suggest enlarging or impending rupture of a thoracic aorta.

Aortography is essential in providing proper diagnosis and precise information regarding the location of the aneurysm. This will indicate the proper surgical approach. Direct arterial injection of contrast material, using a retrograde catheter technique, provides the best information. In addition, concomitant left-heart catheterization or coronary arteriograms can be performed when indicated. Usually, the aneurysm is identified. However, if the aneurysm is filled with laminated thrombus, the lumen may appear to be relatively normal. In most instances, the width of the arterial wall can be determined. A characteristic double lumen, showing a true and false lumen, is usually seen in dissecting aneurysms. The true lumen may be compressed or distorted, and it may not be possible to detect branches, as they are occluded by dissection.

MEDICAL AND SURGICAL TREATMENT

We believe that the majority of patients with thoracic aortic aneurysms should be treated surgically. Medical therapy is indicated during diagnosis, stabilization of the patient's condition, preparation for surgical management and for control of associated illnesses. Medical treatment of acute dissecting aneurysms is directed to control of hypertension and reduction of cardiac contractility. This usually stabilizes the acute dissection and allows elective surgical intervention. Emergency surgical intervention is required when there is evidence that the aneurysm has ruptured or is about to rupture. Traumatic lacerations of the aorta obviously require immediate surgical intervention. Acute dissecting aneurysms should be operated on if the patient's condition cannot be controlled medically. Continued pain, impending rupture, occlusion of a major branch of the aorta, severe aortic valvular incompetence, or cardiac tamponade are indications for emergency operation. The surgical procedure will vary according to the location and the extent of the aneurysm.

Aneurysms of the
Ascending Aorta

The surgical approach is through a median sternotomy. The operation is performed using total cardiopulmonary bypass (Figure 2). The arterial cannula from the pump oxygenator is placed in the common femoral artery. The venous cannulae are usually inserted through the right atrium into the inferior and superior venae cavae. If the aneurysm is large, or if dense adhesions make cannulization difficult, then the inferior vena cava catheter can be placed through the common femoral vein. After instituting partial cardiopulmonary bypass, the superior vena cava catheter can more safely be introduced through the right atrium. A cannula is inserted into the left

ventricle at the junction of the left atrium and right superior pulmonary vein, and introduced through the left atrium into the left ventricle via the mitral valve.

The ascending aorta is clamped distal to the aneurysm and just proximal to the innominate artery. A longitudinal aortotomy is made and coronary perfusion is instituted. The diseased intima and media are removed, leaving the surrounding outer layer intact.

Resection of the aortic valve with prosthetic valve replacement or repair of the aortic valve is indicated if there is concomitant aortic valvular disease. The distal ascending aorta

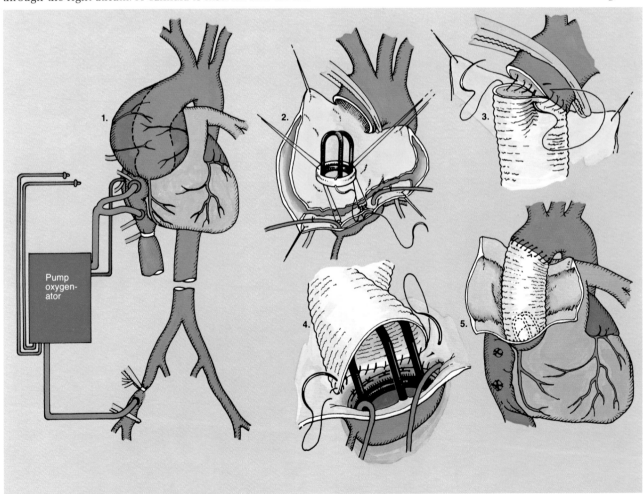

Figure 2. Steps in operative correction of patient with dissecting aneurysm of ascending aorta with aortic valvular insufficiency. Operation is performed under total cardiopulmonary bypass with coronary artery perfusion. The aneurysm of the ascending aorta is resected and replaced with a woven Dacron tube, and the aortic valve is resected and replaced with a ball valve aortic prosthesis.

Aneurysms of the Transverse Arch

is trimmed and an end-to-end anastomosis performed to the distal end of a woven Dacron tube graft. The proximal suture anastomosis is done in a similar manner. Just before completion of the proximal anastomosis, the sump suction is stopped and the caval tourniquets are released, allowing the heart to fill with blood. This enables trapped air to escape. The coronary perfusion catheters are removed and the proximal aortic anastomosis is completed. An additional venting needle is placed near the proximal aortic anastomosis to remove residual air. The distal aortic clamp is gradually released. Additional interrupted sutures with Dacron pledgets, to prevent tearing of the aortic wall, are used if necessary to control anastomotic leaks. The sump and caval catheters are removed. Anticoagulation with heparin is reversed by administration of protamine sulfate. The outer wall of the aneurysm is sutured around the graft, and the pericardium can be closed loosely. Drainage tubes are inserted and the chest is closed.

If there is a well-localized sacciform aneurysm, resection and replacement with a patch aortoplasty may be used instead of replacement with a tube graft. Also, if a dissection of the aorta is encountered, the false lumen must be obliterated before the graft is sutured.

During surgery for aneurysms of the transverse arch (Figure 3), special consideration must be given to providing cerebral arterial perfusion. Resection is carried out through a median sternotomy. In addition to placing the standard cannulae in the femoral artery, in the superior and inferior venae cavae via a right atriotomy, and a left ventricular sump, it is necessary to cannulate the right and left axillary arteries and the left common carotid arteries. This provides circulation to the brain during subsequent cardiopulmonary bypass.

The operative procedure is as follows:

Occluding clamps are applied distal to the aneurysm and to the innominate, left carotid, and left subclavian arteries.

The aneurysm is incised longitudinally, and coronary perfusion is then established. The diseased intima, debris, and laminated thrombus material are removed.

Proximal and distal aortic segments are trimmed, and an appropriate-sized woven Dacron graft is selected.

Distal anastomosis is performed, followed by the proximal anastomosis.

As the coronary perfusion catheters are removed, the left ventricular sump is terminated and the caval catheters are released, allowing blood to fill the heart and evacuate air.

Cardiac function is allowed to resume, restoring circulation through the graft.

Perfusion through the brachiocephalic vessels is continued until continuity of flow to these vessels has been reestablished from the aortic graft – accomplished by anastomosing these vessels individually, either as a cuff or with a separate interposition of woven Dacron tube graft between the vessels and the aortic graft.

End-to-side aortic anastomosis is carried out by applying a partially occluding clamp.

Distal anastomoses to the innominate, left carotid, and left subclavian arteries are established in an end-to-end fashion.

When circulation has been reestablished through the arch vessels, the pump oxygenator is discontinued.

Perfusion cannulae to the brachiocephalic vessels are removed and heparinization is reversed.

Finally, the wound is closed.

102

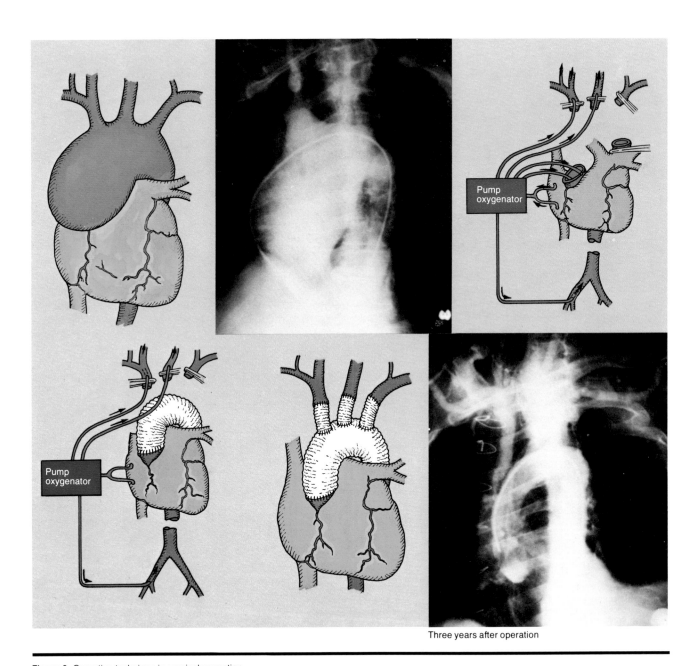

Three years after operation

Figure 3. Operative technique in surgical correction of an aneurysm of the arch of the aorta, using total cardiopulmonary bypass with coronary artery bypass. A three-year postoperative angiogram demonstrates the patent grafts.

Aneurysms of the Descending Thoracic Aorta

Dissecting Aneurysms

Aneurysms of the descending thoracic aorta are approached through a posterior lateral left thoracotomy incision (Figure 4). The selection of the intercostal space depends on the location of the aneurysm; usually the fifth intercostal space provides adequate exposure. Transsection of the posterior upper and lower adjacent ribs provides more exposure.

When the aneurysm has been exposed, the proximal aortic clamp is applied and systemic heparinization, without left atrial-femoral artery bypass, is used. The distal clamp is applied. Palpation of the left carotid artery by the anesthesiologist will ensure that this vessel has not been compromised by the proximal clamp. The outer wall of the aneurysm is incised, and the laminated clot, debris, and intima are removed. Bleeding intercostal arteries are suture ligated. A woven Dacron tube graft of appropriate size is selected and end-to-end proximal and then distal anastomoses are carried out. Before the distal anastomosis is completed, the proximal and distal segments are flushed. Then the distal clamp is removed, evacuating the air and allowing the graft to fill with blood. The proximal clamp is released slowly to avoid hypotension.

Paraplegia, secondary to spinal cord ischemia, is the major complication related to the resection of the descending thoracic aorta. Various attempts have been made in the past to minimize spinal cord ischemia, including left atrial to femoral artery bypass or femoral vein to femoral artery bypass, with the pump oxygenator. With these techniques, the incidence of paraplegia has been reduced to 3% to 4%. Recent experience has shown that aneurysms can be resected successfully without using distal perfusion and without increasing the incidence of neurological complications. This technique has the added advantage of minimizing postoperative pulmonary contusion and congestion. Without distal perfusion, the operative time is reduced and there is less blood loss.

Dissecting aneurysms (Figure 5) are treated essentially by the same method of resection described previously. The exception is that care must be given to the false lumen. After the ascending or descending thoracic aorta has been divided, the proximal and distal ends of the false lumen are obliterated by continuous suture. Graft replacement is then performed. Aortic valve replacement is performed if necessary.

RESULTS OF TREATMENT

During the past 20 years, improvements in diagnosis, surgical technique, and postoperative care have significantly reduced mortality associated with surgical treatment for aneurysms of the thoracic aorta. The operative mortality for patients with aneurysms of the ascending and descending thoracic aorta is 8% to 12%; it is about 15% for aneurysms of the transverse arch. Surgical risk is increased for patients with hypertension or coronary artery disease. Our follow-up studies (extending for as long as 20 years) have revealed the following: (1) postoperative complications have been reduced and long-term survival can be expected; (2) the most common cause of death after operation is concomitant coronary artery disease; (3) the treatment of choice is early recognition and proper surgical management for patients with aneurysms of the thoracic aorta.

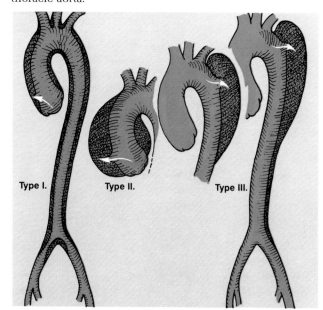

Figure 5. Classification of dissecting aneurysms of the aorta.

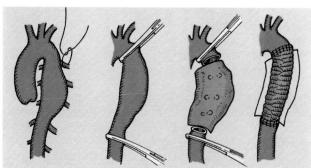

Figure 4. Operative technique for resection of fusiform aneurysm of descending thoracic aorta without bypass, and replacement with woven Dacron tube graft.

Aneurysms of the Thoracoabdominal Aorta

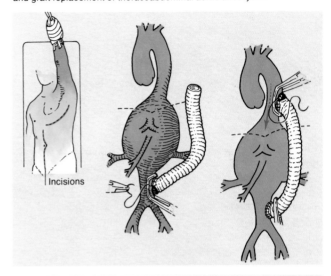

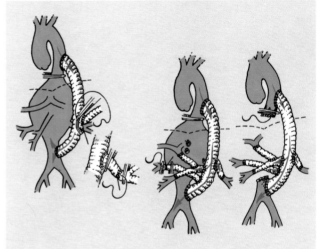

Patients with aneurysms involving the upper segment of the abdominal aorta present another serious and very challenging surgical problem. These aneurysms often extend proximally through the diaphragm and involve the descending thoracic aorta. The complicating factor is that the arterial blood supply to the major visceral organs arises from this segment of the aorta. There is always the potential danger of irreversible ischemia in one or more of the visceral organs. Patients with such aneurysms usually have a pulsatile mass high in the epigastrium. They may have abdominal or back pain, associated symptoms of chronic mesenteric insufficiency, or hypertension related to renal vascular ischemia.

There are two major considerations for resection and graft replacement of aneurysms of the thoracoabdominal segment. The first is to provide adequate exposure of the lesion as well as of normal arterial segments above and below the aneurysm; the second – *and most important* – is to protect the gastrointestinal tract, liver, and kidneys from ischemic damage during surgery.

SURGICAL TECHNIQUE

The patient is positioned on the operating table and a midline incision is made to expose the peritoneal cavity (Figure 6). The abdominal aorta is thoroughly explored first, to determine the extent of the aneurysm. The distal abdominal aorta below the aneurysm is then exposed, and a woven Dacron tube graft is attached, using end-to-side anastomosis and a partially occluding clamp. If the aneurysm or associated occlusive disease extends to the bifurcation of the aorta, each limb of a bifurcation graft is attached by an end-to-side anastomosis to the iliac vessels. The graft is then occluded at its origin, maintaining normal blood flow to the extremities. The left pleural cavity is entered through an anterolateral left thoracotomy incision, usually via the seventh intercostal space. The descending thoracic aorta is exposed proximal to the aneurysm. The previously attached graft is tunneled through the left retroperitoneal gutter, through the diaphragm near the aortic hiatus, and into the pleural cavity. The partially occluding clamp is applied to the distal descending thoracic aorta above the aneurysm, and the previously inserted graft is anastomosed end-to-side. The partially occluding clamp is removed, and blood is routed through the thoracoabdominal bypass graft by occluding the descending thoracic aorta distal to the proximal anastomosis. Appropriate-sized knitted Dacron grafts are attached to the thoraco-

abdominal graft, using an end-to-side anastomosis and a partially occluding clamp. These grafts are then attached individually to each renal artery, to the superior mesenteric artery, and subsequently to the celiac artery, using an end-to-end anastomosis.

With this technique, the ischemic time for each visceral branch is limited to the period of time required for one anastomosis. Following restoration of circulation to the renal, superior mesenteric, and celiac arteries, the aneurysm can be resected and the bed oversewn to control hemorrhage. The ends of the resected thoracic and abdominal aortas are oversewn. The wounds are then closed.

The operative mortality for this extended operation is approximately 15%. If the patient survives the immediate postoperative period, long-term patency of grafts has generally been observed. Studies of renal, hepatic, and gastrointestinal function, years after operation, have shown sustained normal function.

Aneurysms of the Abdominal Aorta

The most common location of aneurysmal disease is in the abdominal aorta. One of the most serious of all diseases, it may result in rupture and death if not diagnosed early. Without surgical treatment, about one half of patients die of rupture within one year after diagnosis; 91% die within five years of diagnosis. The low incidence of surgical mortality has provided an alternative approach for managing these patients, and long-term survival is expected. Thus, except in unusual circumstances, surgery has evolved as the treatment of choice.

Abdominal aortic aneurysms occur in patients of all ages. However, the greatest incidence is reported among older patients, and approximately 20% of the patients are more than 70 years old. The ratio of men to women is about nine to one. Concomitant aortic-iliac occlusive vascular disease, hypertension, cerebrovascular insufficiency, or coronary artery disease may also be present.

Sometimes the abdominal aortic aneurysm may not produce symptoms and is detected only by palpation on routine physical examination, or incidentally with roentgenograms of the abdomen. In other cases, the patient may be aware of a prominent aortic pulsation, or he may experience pain caused by a pathological change in the wall of the aneurysm, such as expansion, leakage, or rupture. The location and severity of pain are dependent upon the nature and extent of these pathological changes. The pain may be localized in the back or may radiate into the flanks, groin, testicle, or leg. If the aneurysm ruptures, the patient develops tachycardia, syncope, diaphoresis, severe pain, and hypotension, and may expire without surgical intervention.

DIAGNOSTIC TECHNIQUES

The usual physical finding is a pulsatile mass in the mid or upper abdomen just to the left of the midline. Tenderness may be present. If leakage or rupture has occurred, there also may be signs of peritoneal irritation, hypotension, sweating, stupor, or oliguria.

Plain roentgenograms of the abdomen in the anteroposterior and lateral projections are particularly helpful in confirming the diagnosis. A ring of calcification in the aneurysmal wall or an area of increased density in the region of the suspected aneurysm is suggestive of an abdominal aortic aneurysm.

Aortography is indicated, however, if one suspects associated occlusive disease of the renal or iliac arteries, or considers the possibility of suprarenal involvement. Because intraluminal thrombi form less frequently in the suprarenal aorta, aneurysms in this location are more clearly defined by aortography. However, aortography may not reveal a widened lumen, because the intraluminal space in the usual variety of infrarenal aortic aneurysm is filled with laminated clot, and the effective luminal size is normal.

Many patients with aneurysms of the abdominal aorta have associated atherosclerotic disease in other organs. Approximately one fourth of the patients have coronary artery disease, and one third have a history of hypertension. Many patients have associated cerebrovascular insufficiency, peripheral vascular occlusive disease, aneurysms of the thoracic aorta, or diabetes. If a patient has aneurysms of both the thoracic and the abdominal aortas, it is usually preferable to resect the abdominal aorta first. The time of convalescence from resection of abdominal aortic aneurysm is shorter, often making it possible to resect the descending thoracic aortic aneurysm during the same hospitalization. Most aneurysms of the infrarenal abdominal aorta are fusiform; sacciform aneurysms are rare. However, associated aneurysmal disease of the iliac vessels may be observed.

SURGICAL TREATMENT

Surgery is recommended once a definitive diagnosis is made. The aneurysm is approached through an extended midline abdominal incision (Figure 7). The retroperitoneal space is opened and the aortic aneurysm is exposed. In most cases, a satisfactory cuff of abdominal aorta is present below the renal arteries. Distal dissection can be carried out until a relatively normal segment of distal abdominal aorta or iliac artery is encountered. The proximal aortic clamp is applied below the renal arteries after introduction of intra-arterial heparin. A longitudinal aortotomy is made, incising the outer wall of the aneurysm. Blunt dissection is completed in the posterior direction. The laminated clot, diseased intima, and debris are then removed. The lumbar arteries are sutured. An appropriate-sized woven Dacron graft is selected. A straight tube graft may be used if the aneurysm is confined to the abdominal aorta and the aortic bifurcation is relatively normal. A bifurcation graft is used if the aneurysmal disease extends into the iliac arteries or if there is concomitant occlusive disease. The proximal end-to-end anastomosis is accomplished. The distal anastomosis can be carried out, either to the terminal abdominal aorta at the bifurcation, or to the common iliac arteries in an end-to-end fashion. If there is

106

associated occlusive disease, an end-to-side anastomosis can be performed to the external iliac artery within the abdominal cavity. The aortic clamp is released slowly to avoid hypotension. Usually, the inferior mesenteric artery is small and easily ligated. If, however, the inferior mesenteric artery is large and provides significant collateral circulation to the bowel, this artery may be preserved with a button of aortic tissue and resutured to the abdominal aortic graft. If the patient has associated renovascular hypertension, appropriate side grafts can be made from the abdominal aortic graft to the renal artery. After completion of the graft replacement, the retroperitoneal space is approximated and the wound is closed.

Surgical resection for treatment of abdominal aortic aneurysms has proven to be one of the most effective advances in peripheral vascular surgery. The operative mortality has been

reduced to approximately 3%. However, increased mortality may be expected in patients with severe coronary artery disease or hypertension. Long-term studies reveal approximately 60% survival after five years. Another major factor influencing early mortality and long-term survival is the condition of the aneurysm at the time of resection. If the aneurysm has leaked or ruptured, mortality may be as high as 30% to 50%. Age has not been found to be a contraindication for surgical treatment. With proper surgical management and good postoperative care, older patients have an excellent prognosis.

Aneurysms may also be seen in other peripheral arteries, such as the femoral, popliteal, carotid, and subclavian arteries. Splanchnic artery aneurysms involving the mesenteric or renal arteries are less common. These, too, can be treated successfully with surgical excision and graft replacement.

Figure 7. Technique of excision and graft replacement of abdominal aortic aneurysm involving distal aorta and common iliac arteries.

a. Incision
b. Aneurysm opened, thrombus and intima removed
c. Lumbar arteries ligated, and proximal aorta trimmed
d. Proximal anastomosis performed
e. Left limb of graft anastomosed to left iliac artery
f. Graft flushed, clamp placed on right limb, and anastomosis performed
g. Clamps removed, peritoneum and remaining aneurysmal wall closed over graft

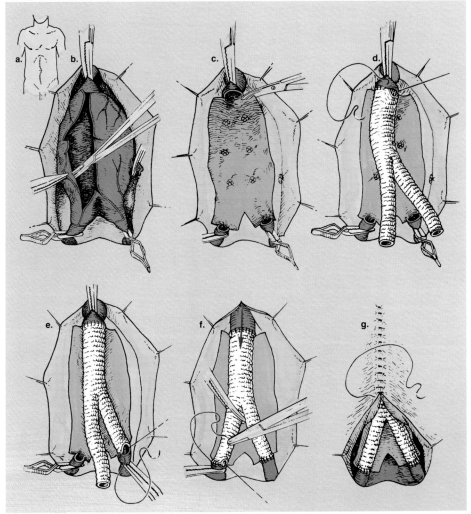

ACKNOWLEDGMENTS

The following figures have been reproduced by permission of the authors and publishers.

Figure 1. DeBakey ME, Beall AC Jr: Surgical treatment of diseases of the aorta and major arteries, in Hurst WJ, Logue RB (eds): *The Heart,* ed 2, 1970, p 1527. Courtesy of McGraw-Hill Book Co Inc, New York, NY.

Figure 3. DeBakey ME, Beall AC Jr, Cooley DA, et al: Resection and graft replacement of aneurysms involving the transverse arch of the aorta. *Surg Clin North Am* 46:1060, 1966. Courtesy WB Saunders Co, Philadelphia, PA.

Figure 5. DeBakey ME, Beall AC Jr, Cooley DA, et al: Dissecting aneurysms of the aorta. *Surg Clin North Am* 46:1046, 1966. Courtesy WB Saunders Co, Philadelphia, PA.

Figures 6A and 6B. Garrett HE, Crawford ES, Beall AC Jr, et al: Surgical treatment of aneurysm of the thoracoabdominal aorta. *Surg Clin North Am* 46:915, 1966. Courtesy WB Saunders Co, Philadelphia, PA.

Figure 7. Crawford ES, DeBakey ME, Morris GC Jr, et al: Aneurysm of the abdominal aorta. *Surg Clin North Am* 46:975, 1966. Courtesy WB Saunders Co, Philadelphia, PA.

Supplementary Reading

Section I
Antonio M. Gotto, Jr., MD

Dawber TR: Risk factors for atherosclerotic disease. A Scope® monograph, Kalamazoo, The Upjohn Co, 1975.

Dustan HP: Vascular diseases of hypertension. *Atherosclerosis Revs*, to be published.

Fredrickson DS, Goldstein JL, Brown MS: Familial hyperlipoproteinemia, in Stanbury JB, Wyngaarden JB, Fredrickson DS (eds): *The Metabolic Basis of Inherited Disease*. New York, McGraw Hill, to be published.

Jackson RL, Morrisett JD, Gotto AM Jr: Lipoprotein structure and metabolism. *Physiol Rev* 56:259-316, 1976.

Clofibrate and niacin in coronary disease, Coronary Drug Project Research Group. *JAMA* 237 (4): 360, 1975.

Keys A: Coronary heart disease – the global picture. *Atherosclerosis 22*: 149-192, 1975.

Laragh JH (ed): *Hypertension manual*, ed 1. Dun–Donnelley Publishing Corp, 1975.

Executive summary of the task force reports to the Hypertension Information and Education Advisory Committee, National High Blood Pressure Education Program. Bethesda, National Institutes of Health, 1973, pp 1-20.

Stamler J, Berkson DM, Lindberg HA: Risk factors: Their roles in the etiology and pathogenesis of the atherosclerotic diseases, in Wissler RW, Geer JC (eds): *The Pathogenesis of Atherosclerosis*. Baltimore, Williams & Wilkins, 1972, p 41.

Yeshurun D, Gotto AM: Drug treatment of hyperlipidemia. *Am J Med* 60:379-393, 1976.

Section II
Abel Lazzarini Robertson, Jr., MD

Benditt EP: Evidence for a monoclonal origin of human atherosclerotic plaques and some implications. *Circulation* 50:650, 1974.

Brown MS, Goldstein JL: Regulation of the activity of the low-density lipoprotein receptor in human fibroblasts. *Cell* 6:307, 1975.

Geer JC: Fine structure of human aortic intimal thickening and fatty streaks. *Lab Invest* 14:1764, 1965.

Geer JC, Glagov S, Haust MD, et al: Relationship of hypertension to vascular changes: II. Atherosclerosis, in Page IH, McCubbin J (eds): *Renal Hypertension*. Chicago, Yearbook Medical Publishers, 1968, pp 385-390.

Haust MD, More RH: Development of modern theories on the pathogenesis of atherosclerosis, in Wissler RW, Geer JC (eds): *The Pathogenesis of Atherosclerosis*. Baltimore, Williams & Wilkins, 1972, pp 1-16.

Kritchevsky D, Kothari, HV: Metabolism of the arterial wall, in Schettler G, Weizel A (eds): *Atherosclerosis III*. Berlin, Heidelberg, New York, Springer-Verlag, 1974, pp 39-45.

McGill HC: The lesion, in Schettler G, Weizel A (eds): *Atherosclerosis III*. Berlin, Heidelberg, New York, Springer-Verlag, 1974, pp 27-37.

McMillan GD: Development of arteriosclerosis. *Am J Cardiol* 31:542, 1973.

More RH: Definition of early human lesions, morphology and histochemistry, in Schettler G, Weizel A (eds): *Atherosclerosis III*. Berlin, Heidelberg, New York, Springer-Verlag, 1974, pp 1-2.

Mustard JF, Packham MA: Thrombosis and the development of atherosclerosis, in Wissler RW, Geer JC (eds): *The Pathogenesis of Atherosclerosis*. Baltimore, Williams & Wilkins, 1972, pp 214-226.

Pesonen E, Norio R, Sarna S: Thickenings in the coronary arteries in infancy as an indication of genetic factors in coronary heart disease. *Circulation 51*: 218, 1975.

Roberts WC: Coronary artery pathology in fatal ischemic heart disease, in Braunwald E (ed): *The Myocardium: Failure and Infarction*. New York, HP Publishing Co, 1974, pp 192-204.

Robertson AL Jr: Transport of plasma lipoproteins and ultrastructure of human arterial intimacytes in culture, in Rothblat GH, Kritchevsky D (eds): *Lipid Metabolism in Tissue Culture Cells, The Wistar Symposium Monograph No. 6*. Philadelphia, The Wistar Institute Press, 1967, pp 115-128.

Robertson AL Jr, Khairallah PA: Arterial endothelial permeability and vascular disease: The "trap door" effect. *Exp Mol Pathol* 18:241, 1973.

Robertson AL Jr: Functional characterization of arterial cells involved in spontaneous atheroma, in Schettler G, Weizel A (eds): *Atherosclerosis III*. Berlin, Springer-Verlag, 1974, pp 175-184.

Ross R: The arterial smooth-muscle cell, in Wissler RW, Geer JC (eds): *The Pathogenesis of Atherosclerosis*. Baltimore, Williams & Wilkins, 1972, pp 147-163.

Stehbens WE: Cerebral atherosclerosis: Intimal proliferation and atherosclerosis in the cerebral arteries. *Arch Pathol* 99:582, 1975.

Stein Y, Stein O: Lipid synthesis and degradation and lipoprotein transport in mammalian aorta, in *Atherogenesis, Initiating Factors*. Ciba Foundation Symposium 12, Amsterdam, 1973, pp 165-183.

Tejada C, Strong JP, Montenegro MR, et al: Distribution of coronary and aortic atherosclerosis by geographic location, race and sex. *Lab Invest 18*: 509, 1968.

Wissler RW: Development of the atherosclerotic plaque, in Braunwald E (ed): *The Myocardium: Failure and Infarction*. New York, HP Publishing Co, 1974, pp 155-166.

Sections III and IV
Stephen E. Epstein, MD

Epstein SE, Redwood DR, Goldstein RE, et al: Angina pectoris: Pathophysiology, evaluation, and treatment. *Ann Intern Med 75*:263-296, 1971.

Redwood DR, Epstein SE: The uses and limitations of stress testing in the evaluation of ischemic heart disease. *Circulation 46*:1115-1131, 1972.

Borer JS, Brensike JF, Redwood DR, et al: Limitations of the electrocardiographic response to exercise in predicting coronary-artery disease. *N Engl J Med 293*:367-371, 1975.

Strauss HW, Pitt B, James AE Jr (eds); *Cardiovascular Nuclear Medicine.* St. Louis, CV Mosby, 1974.

Index

114